American Medical Association Contact Information

American Medical Association
515 N State St, Chicago, IL 60654   (312) 464-5000
www.ama-assn.org

Membership information
(800) 262-3211   *msc@ama-assn.org*
www.ama-assn.org/go/membership

Adolescent health
(312) 464-5315   *gaps@ama-assn.org*
www.ama-assn.org/go/adolescenthealth

Allied health education
(312) 464-4635   *fred.lenhoff@ama-assn.org*
www.ama-assn.org/go/alliedhealth

AMA Foundation
(312) 464-4200   *steven.churchill@ama-assn.org*
www.amafoundation.org

Becoming a Physician
becominganmd@ama-assn.org
www.ama-assn.org/go/becominganmd

Continuing medical education
(312) 464-4671   *cme@ama-assn.org*
www.ama-assn.org/go/cme

Council on Ethical and Judicial Affairs
(312) 464-4823   *ceja@ama-assn.org*
www.ama-assn.org/go/ceja

Council on Medical Education
(312) 464-4515   *daniel.winship@ama-assn.org*
www.ama-assn.org/go/councilmeded

Council on Science and Public Health
(312) 464-5046   *csaph@ama-assn.org*
www.ama-assn.org/go/csa

Domestic violence
(312) 464-5376   *violence@ama-assn.org*
www.ama-assn.org/go/violence

Find a residency or fellowship
(312) 464-4748   *rfs@ama-assn.org*
www.ama-assn.org/go/rfs

FREIDA Online
(800) 266-3966   *freida@ama-assn.org*
www.ama-assn.org/go/freida

Genetics and molecular medicine
(312) 464-4964   *srt@ama-assn.org*
www.ama-assn.org/go/genetics

Gifts to physicians from industry
(312) 464-4668   *cppd@ama-assn.org*
www.ama-assn.org/go/ethicalgifts

GME data requests
(312) 464-4487   *sarah.brotherton@ama-assn.org*

GME Directory
(312) 464-4635   *fred.lenhoff@ama-assn.org*
www.ama-assn.org/go/mededproducts

GME e-Letter
(312) 464-4635   *gme@ama-assn.org*
www.ama-assn.org/go/gmenews

GME program director mailing labels
(312) 464-4635   *fred.lenhoff@ama-assn.org*

Health disparities
(312) 464-4616   *tanya.lopez@ama-assn.org*
www.ama-assn.org/go/enddisparities

Health literacy
(312) 464-5357   *louella.hung@ama-assn.org*
www.amafoundation.org

Infectious Diseases
(312) 464-4147
www.ama-assn.org/go/infectiousdiseases

Liaison Committee on Medical Education
(312) 464-4690   *barbara.barzansky@ama-assn.org*
www.lcme.org

Medical education books and CDs
(312) 464-4635   *fred.lenhoff@ama-assn.org*
www.ama-assn.org/go/mededproducts

Medical Education Bulletin
(312) 464-4693   *sylvia.etzel@ama-assn.org*

Medical licensure
(312) 464-4635   *fred.lenhoff@ama-assn.org*
www.ama-assn.org/go/licensure

National GME Census
(800) 866-6793   *gmetrack@aamc.org*
www.aamc.org/gmetrack

State-level GME data
(312) 464-4659   *jacqueline.edwards@ama-assn.org*

Virtual Mentor
(312) 464-5260   *virtualmentor@ama-assn.org*
www.virtualmentor.org

AMA Sections/Interest Groups; AMA Advocacy Agenda

The AMA represents you: Join today

The AMA offers many sections and special groups representing all physicians. All members receive the *Journal of the American Medical Association* and *American Medical News*. To join the AMA, call (800) AMA-3211, access *www.ama-assn.org/go/join*, or complete the enclosed membership form.

Gay, Lesbian, Bisexual and Transgender (GLBT) Issues Advisory Committee
(312) 464-4748   *glbt@ama-assn.org*
www.ama-assn.org/go/glbt

Group Practice Physicians Advisory Committee
(312) 464-4546   *carrie.waller@ama-assn.org*
www.ama-assn.org/go/medicalgroup

International Medical Graduate Section
(312) 464-5678   *img@ama-assn.org*
www.ama-assn.org/go/imgs

Medical Student Section
(312) 464-4746   *mss@ama-assn.org*
www.ama-assn.org/go/mss

Minority Affairs Consortium
(312) 464-4335   *mac@ama-assn.org*
www.ama-assn.org/go/mac

Organized Medical Staff Section
(312) 464-2461   *omss@ama-assn.org*
www.ama-assn.org/go/omss

Resident and Fellow Section
(312) 464-4748   *rfs@ama-assn.org*
www.ama-assn.org/go/rfs

Section on Medical Schools
(312) 464-4655   *section@ama-assn.org*
www.ama-assn.org/go/sms

Senior Physicians Group
(312) 464-4539   *spg@ama-assn.org*
www.ama-assn.org/go/spg

Women Physicians Congress
(312) 464-4335   *wpc@ama-assn.org*
www.ama-assn.org/go/wpc

Young Physicians Section
(312) 464-4751   *yps@ama-assn.org*
www.ama-assn.org/go/yps

AMA National Health Care Policy Agenda

The AMA believes that all Americans are worthy of a fair and affordable health system. Today, Americans are faced with a fragmented health system. Millions don't visit a doctor until their illness reaches a serious stage. As a nation, we can and should do better.

At the center of the AMA's vision is the concept that every American, regardless of means, has health insurance, and every patient maintains the freedom to choose his or her own doctors and health plans and maintains control over his or her own care. Specifically:

- The AMA urges lawmakers to implement a system of tax credits to enable individuals to buy health insurance. We have a detailed proposal for this system.

- Under current law, Medicare will make deep cuts in payments to doctors every year until 2015. This policy erodes patient access to care and is a barrier to practice innovations. Congress and the Administration need to permanently replace the flawed payment formula.

- Medical lawsuits are driving up health costs for everyone and making it hard for many to find a doctor. The AMA seeks reasonable limits on the noneconomic damages juries can award so that doctors aren't forced to move, cut services, or go out of business.

Physicians and other health providers must work with government and private payers on strategies to restrain rising health care costs while maintaining quality of care. Medical science and technology have moved forward at a lightning pace. Patients are ready for the American health system to follow suit. The AMA is committed to:

- Finding new ways to enable doctors to use promising new technology

- Pioneering new methods to measure and improve the quality of care

- Preventing errors by studying ones that have happened, without the threat of lawsuits

- Directing more resources and effort toward disease prevention

- Helping Americans lead more healthful lifestyles

- Eliminating gaps in care, particularly for racial and ethnic minority patients, the elderly, and low-income families

- Preparing better for large-scale health care emergencies

Our nation needs a well-trained medical workforce, and more doctors, particularly in physician shortage/underserved areas and in undersupplied specialties. We must make sure our medical education stays the best in the world, and make paying for it less burdensome. So too must we address the barriers that threaten the viability of many physician practices, such as:

- Payments that do not reflect the true cost of providing care

- Health insurers' deceptive business practices

- Antitrust rules that restrict doctors from negotiating with health insurance companies

As physicians and medical students, we see firsthand every day how urgently our patients need a better health system. Together, we can shape one America truly deserves.

Visit *www.ama-assn.org/go/agenda* to learn more.

Medical Licensure and Medical Education Organizations

Accreditation Council for Graduate Medical Education (ACGME)
515 N State St
Chicago, IL 60654
(312) 755-5000   (312) 755-7498 Fax
www.acgme.org

American Board of Medical Specialties (ABMS)
222 N LaSalle St, Ste 1500
Chicago, IL 60601
(312) 436-2600
www.abms.org

American Hospital Association (AHA)
One N Franklin
Chicago, IL 60606
(312) 422-3000   (312) 422-4796 Fax
www.aha.org

Educational Commission for Foreign Medical Graduates (ECFMG)
3624 Market Street
Philadelphia, PA 19104-2685
(215) 386-5900   (215) 386-9196 Fax
www.ecfmg.org

Federation of Medical Regulatory Authorities of Canada
2283 St Laurent Blvd, Ste 103
Ottawa, ON K1G 5A2
(613) 738-0372   (613) 738-9169 Fax
www.fmrac.ca

Federation of State Medical Boards (FSMB)
PO Box 619850
Dallas, TX 75261-9850
(817) 868-4000   (817) 868-4099 Fax
www.fsmb.org

The Joint Commission
One Renaissance Blvd
Oakbrook Terrace, IL 60181
(630) 792-5000   (630) 792-5005 Fax
www.jointcommission.org

National Board of Medical Examiners (NBME)
3750 Market St
Philadelphia, Pa 19104-3102
(215) 590-9500   (215) 590-9555 Fax
www.nbme.org

National Board of Osteopathic Medical Examiners (NBOME)
8765 W Higgins Rd, Ste 200
Chicago, IL 60631-4101
(773) 714-0622   (773) 714-0631 Fax
www.nbome.org

National Committee for Quality Assurance (NCQA)
1100 13th St, NW
Washington, DC 20056
(202) 955-3500   (202) 955-3599 Fax
www.ncqa.org

National Practitioner Data Bank and Healthcare Integrity and Protection Data Bank
PO Box 10832
Chantilly, VA 20153-0832
(800) 767-6732
www.npdb-hipdb.com

Royal College of Physicians and Surgeons of Canada
774 Echo Dr
Ottawa, Ontario, K1S 5N8
(800) 668-3740   (613) 730-8830 Fax
http://rcpsc.medical.org

United States Medical Licensing Examination (USMLE)
3750 Market St
Philadelphia, PA 19104-3190
(215) 590-9700   (215) 590-9470 Fax
www.usmle.org

Assessing medical education and career options?

Beginning a residency or practice?

Considering a career change?

Determining whether to relocate or retire?

The AMA wrote the book—in fact, more than a dozen books—to help you with the ABCs (and even Ds!) of medical education and practice. See "Helpful Practice Management Resources From the AMA" on the next page.

Helpful Practice Management Resources From the AMA

Compliance Guide for the Medical Practice: How to Attain and Maintain a Compliant Medical Practice

This resource contains extensive information and instructions on creating a compliance program to help safeguard your practice from risk, both legal and financial. Topics include billing and reimbursement compliance, personnel policies, OSHA, CLIA, and HIPAA. Checklists and practical guidelines are included to help evaluate your practice and train staff to develop, implement, and maintain compliance programs.
OP312006   Price: $99.95 (AMA member price: $74.95)

The Physician's Guide to Survival and Success in the Medical Practice

This invaluable reference guide, which details the day-to-day operation of a medical practice, offers practical tools and techniques for successfully managing personnel, finance and operations, marketing and promotion, and risk. Up-to-date coverage of electronic health records and other technologies are also included. Presented in an easy-to-use three-ring binder format, this resource provides numerous forms as well as evaluation and assessment tools. Additional aids are provided on the CD-ROM.
OP401607   Price: $135 (AMA member price: $105)

Maximizing Billing and Collections in the Medical Practice

Learn a systematic approach to reviewing your billing and collections process to help discover problems and prevent undue financial losses. Given today's shrinking physician reimbursement environment, practices need the right tools and information to maximize their billing and collections efforts—this book helps physicians do just that. Includes CD-ROM with additional tools and content.
OP318607   Price: $75.95 (AMA member price: $56.95)

A Guide to Patient Safety

Gain a comprehensive understanding of the risks and consequences of errors and adverse events in ambulatory care. Offering an in-depth review, this book begins with a historical perspective of patient safety and the important role it plays today with regard to medical liability, medication dosages, electronic health records, and rules for satisfying patient needs. Includes case studies that provide additional insight into integrating patient safety into the medical practice. Emphasis is also given to creating and incorporating a business model and system support to accomplish your patient safety initiatives.
OP401006   Price: $59.95 (AMA member price: $44.95)

Practical EHR: Electronic Record Solutions for Compliance and Quality Care

The *Practical EHR* approach to electronic records provides physicians and their staff with the knowledge and the tools to take control of the process of investigating, selecting, and implementing an EHR. This book helps medical practices focus on the EHR component that is most critical to physicians—the medical history and physical (H&P). The design and functionality recommendations in this book will help you promote quality care and meet your medical practice's needs.
OP324408   Price: $84.95 (AMA member price: $64.95)

Tools for an Efficient Medical Practice

Designed by the author of the AMA's best-selling *Medical Practice Policies & Procedures* and written from a physician office manager's perspective, this invaluable resource will help physicians and their staff develop a more productive, prosperous medical practice. Content is organized around the use of thoughtfully designed forms, templates and checklists extending to all areas of the medical practice, including administrative, financial, personnel, managed care, marketing, and more. Includes more than 180 customizable forms on CD-ROM to help protect your practice from audit liability while enhancing work flow efficiencies and operations.
OP127108   Price: $64.95 (AMA member price: $49.95)

AMA Physicians' Guide to Financial Planning

All the information physicians need for successful financial planning. Offers solid, common-sense tools tailored to help physicians and their families manage day-to-day financial issues. This interactive guide provides expert advice on financial planning, saving, investing, self-guided portfolio management, obtaining loans and mortgages, buying and selling real estate, retirement, estate planning, and many other aspects of money and investment. Contains worksheets, sample agreements and letters, do-it-yourself formulas, a glossary of terms, and much more.
OP230107   Price: $39.95 (AMA member price: $29.95)

Starting a Medical Practice, Second edition

Whether you're establishing a solo practice or joining a group, beginning the practice of medicine requires considerable forethought. With new and updated information, *Starting a Medical Practice*, Second edition helps physicians ask the right questions before they begin the process, and gives them the business insights they need to get their practices running smoothly from the outset.
OP315202   Price: $55 (AMA member price: $45)

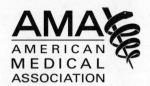

2010 Membership Application

XMBRSP

Yes.

I accept your invitation for a full-year membership in the American Medical Association (AMA).

Members who reside in Mississippi must join directly through the Mississippi State Medical Association.

A physician or medical student who applies for direct membership in the AMA is encouraged to also join his/her state and local medical societies.

Activate your AMA membership today.

Three easy ways:

Call: (800) 262-3211
Fax: (800) 262-3221

Mail:
American Medical Association
Remittance Control
12th floor
515 N State Street
Chicago, IL 60654

If you wish to receive e-mail about AMA advocacy initiatives, news for physicians, and AMA products and services, please add or update your e-mail address below.

My e-mail address is:_____

First name *(please print)*   Middle initial   Last name

Preferred professional mailing address (☐ Home ☐ Office or ☐ Both)

City   State   ZIP

Date of birth *(to aid in tracking/identification)*

Office phone

Fax   Military branch of service

Outreach recruiter name *(if applicable)*

International medical student graduates* *(see back for important information)*

Membership categories and dues rates

Physician

____ $420 Regular practice
____ $315 Second year in medical practice
____ $210 First year in medical practice
____ $280 Military
    (Please indicate branch of service above)
____ $210 Semi-retired
    (65 and over, working 1–20 hours a week)
____ $84 Fully retired
    (Age not withstanding—working 0 hours)

Intern/resident/fellow

____ $45 One-year membership

Up to 11.1% multi-year discount:
____ $160 Four-year membership
____ $120 Three-year membership
____ $80 Two-year membership

Medical student

____ $20 One-year membership

Up to 15% multi-year discount:
____ $68 Four-year membership
____ $54 Three-year membership
____ $38 Two-year membership

Method of payment *(see rate chart above)*

____ Check (Please make your check payable to: American Medical Association)
____ Please charge my: ☐ Visa   ☐ MasterCard   ☐ American Express

Please check credit card payment method below: *(See back for credit card payment information.**)*

Options 1 or 2 below are recommended.

Available to regular, military and fully retired membership categories only.

☐ 1. Single payment with automatic renewal
☐ 2. Installment payments with automatic renewal
☐ 3. Single payment without automatic renewal

Credit card number |_|_|_|_|_|_|_|_|_|_|_|_|_|_|_| Expiration date _____

Cardholder's signature _____

Let us remember for you— choose automatic renewal.

Select automatic renewal and your membership will be reactivated yearly. No more paper dues notices will be sent to you.

Select option 1 or 2

Applying for AMA membership: Membership is contingent upon the American Medical Association's (AMA) acceptance of the membership application. The endorsement, deposit or negotiation of an applicant's check does not guarantee admission into or acceptance of membership by the AMA. Checks received will routinely be deposited without a determination of the propriety of the payment or the applicability of the amount. Applicants who are not admitted to membership will receive a refund from the AMA for the amount submitted.

AMA dues are not deductible as a charitable contribution for federal income tax purposes, but may be partially deducted as a business expense. AMA estimates that 50% of your membership dues are allocable to lobbying activities of the AMA, and therefore are not deductible for income tax purposes.

Dues-paying members are eligible for print copies of *JAMA* and *American Medical News*. For the 2010 membership year, the allocated costs of $33 for *JAMA* and $12 for *American Medical News* are included in, and not deductible from AMA membership dues. All members receive free online access to *JAMA*, *American Medical News* and the *Archives* journals. In addition, all members are eligible for *AMA Morning Rounds*.

International medical student graduates are eligible for AMA membership upon acceptance into an accredited residency or fellowship program in the United States, Puerto Rico, Guam or the Virgin Islands.

Conditions of AMA membership and application: As part of a physician organization committed to strengthening the ethics of medicine, every member pledges to uphold the Principles of Medical Ethics as interpreted in the Code of Medical Ethics, and to comply with the Bylaws of the American Medical Association and the Rules of the AMA Council of Ethical and Judicial Affairs.

- The AMA Principles and the Code of Medical Ethics may be viewed online at: *www.ama-assn.org/go/codeofmedicalethics*

- The AMA's Bylaws and Rules of the Council on Ethical and Judicial Affairs are accessible at: *www.ama-assn.org/go/ceja*

Applicants and members are required to disclose to the AMA Office of General Counsel any violations of the Principles of Medical Ethics or illegal conduct. Additionally, the Health Care Quality Improvement Act requires professional societies (such as the AMA) to report certain professional review actions, including denial of membership, to the National Practitioner Data Bank.

**Credit card payment information:
1. Single payment with automatic renewal is available to regular practice, military and fully retired membership categories only.
2. Installment payment with automatic renewal is available to regular practice, military and fully retired membership categories only.
3. Single payment without automatic renewal is available to all membership categories.

Pay monthly: Installment payments begin with the month payment is received and continue until paid in full by Dec. 31, 2010. Renewal of both automatic payment options will be charged in January 2011, with one lump sum for single payment and 1/12 of the annual fee for installment payments.

Participation in either of the two automatic renewal options ensures continuity of your membership benefits and helps the planet reduce paper waste. With the automatic renewal options, your membership will continue from year to year unless canceled by either party. The AMA will not change your future membership dues without prior written notice.

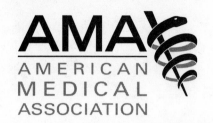

State Medical Licensure Requirements
and Statistics

2010

State Medical Licensure Requirements and Statistics, 2010

Internet address: *www.ama-assn.org*

This book is for informational purposes only. It is not intended to
constitute legal or financial advice. If legal, financial, or other
professional advice is required, the services of a competent
professional should be sought.

Additional copies of this book may be ordered by calling (800) 621-8335
Secure online orders can be taken at *www.amabookstore.com*
Mention product number OP399010

Comments or inquiries
Fred Donini-Lenhoff, Editor
Medical Education Products
American Medical Association
515 North State Street
Chicago, IL 60654
(312) 464-4635
(312) 464-5830 Fax
E-mail: *fred.lenhoff@ama-assn.org*
www.ama-assn.org/go/licensure

ISBN: 978-1-60359-108-9
BP15:09-P-019:10/09

Foreword

State Medical Licensure Requirements and Statistics, 2010, presents current information and statistics on medical licensure in the United States and possessions. Data were obtained from a number of sources, including state boards of medical examiners, the Federation of State Medical Boards, National Board of Medical Examiners, Educational Commission for Foreign Medical Graduates, and the United States Medical Licensing Examination Secretariat.

Licensure data and policies in this publication were compiled from the AMA's 2009 Medical Licensure Survey, which was sent in May 2009 to all 54 allopathic and 14 osteopathic boards of medical examiners in the United States. Although every effort was made to collect and record accurate data for each board, users of this book should note that the boards meet frequently and, as a result, their licensure and examination policies are modified regularly. It is therefore recommended that the state licensing boards (see Appendixes A and B) be contacted for the most up-to-date information.

The following boards did not provide updates to the AMA in 2009 via the licensure survey:

- Connecticut Medical Examining Board
- Guam Board of Medical Examiners
- New Mexico Board of Osteopathic Medical Examiners
- Board of Medical Examiners of Puerto Rico
- Virgin Islands Board of Medical Examiners

For more information

The AMA offers Internet information on medical licensure through its Medical Licensure Online Web site (*www.ama-assn.org/go/licensure*). The site includes information from this book and *Licensing and Credentialing: What Physicians Need to Know*, as well as links to state and national licensing organizations and selected articles on licensure from *American Medical News*.

Acknowledgments

The editor would like to thank the personnel of the state medical and osteopathic licensing agencies who provided statistics and licensing requirements for this publication.

Acknowledgments are also due to the following individuals and organizations for their assistance with updating copy and writing articles:

- Accreditation Council for Continuing Medical Education
  Kate Regnier, MA, MBA
      Deputy Chief Executive

- Accreditation Council for Graduate Medical Education
  Jeanne K. Heard, MD, PhD
      Director, Department of RRC Activities
  Julie Jacob
      Manager of Communications

- Administrators in Medicine
  Barbara Neuman, Executive Director

- American Board of Medical Specialties
  Lori Boukas
      Director of Marketing and Communications
  Sylvia McGreal
      Marketing and Communications Specialist

- Robert D. Aronson, Esq., author of "Immigration Overview for International Medical Graduates"

- Department of the Air Force
  Dale R. Agner, Col, USAF, MC
      Chief, Clinical Quality Management Division
  Kathy A. Smith, CPHQ, CPCS, CPMSM
      Chief, Professional Staff Management

- Department of the Army
  Howard M. Kimes, Colonel, US Army
      Director, Quality Management Directorate
  Janet L. Wilson, Lieutenant Colonel, US Army
      Chief, Regulatory Compliance

- Department of the Navy
  Joseph McBreen, Captain, Medical Corps,
      US Navy Corps, Director, Clinical Operations,
      Bureau of Medicine and Surgery
  Georgi Irvine, Commander, Head, Medical and Dental
      Staff Services, Navy Medical Support Command

- Drug Enforcement Administration, Office of Diversion Control
  Mark W. Caverly, Chief, Liaison and Policy Section

- Educational Commission for Foreign Medical Graduates
  Stephen S. Seeling, JD, Vice President for Operations
  Elizabeth M. Ingraham, Manager, Publications and Special Projects
  Tracy Cuddy
  Administrative Manager, ECFMG Publications

- Federation of Medical Regulatory Authorities of Canada
  Fleur-Ange Lefebvre, Executive Director

- Federation of State Medical Boards of the United States
  Drew Carlson, Director of Communications

- The Joint Commission
  Mark R. Chassin, MD, President
  Ken Powers, Media Relations Manager

- National Board of Medical Examiners and United States Medical Licensing Examination Secretariat
  Kenneth E. Cotton

- National Committee for Quality Assurance
  L. Gregory Pawlson MD, MPH, FACP, Executive Vice President

- National Practitioner Data Bank
  Shirley Jones, JD, MHA, Associate Director

We would also like to acknowledge the contributions of the following AMA staff:

- Division of Survey and Data Resources
  Monica Quiroz, Mark Long, Susan Montrimas, and Derek Smart
- AMA Business Products
  Lori Hollacher, Erin Kalitowski, and JD Kinney
- Medical Education
  Jacqueline Edwards and Gretchen Kenagy, PhD
- Continuing Physician Professional Development
  Jeanette Harmon and Mary Kelly
- Healthcare Education Products and Standards
  R. Mark Evans, PhD, and Patti Fitzgerald

Fred Donini-Lenhoff, Editor

Catherine Welcher, Assistant Editor

Paul H. Rockey, MD, MPH
Director, Division of Graduate Medical Education

Contents

Tables

Section I.

Licensure Policies and Regulations of State Medical/Osteopathic Boards

Administration of the United States Medical Licensing Examination Steps 1 and 2

In 1990, the Federation of State Medical Boards (FSMB) and the National Board of Medical Examiners (NBME) established the United States Medical Licensing Examination (USMLE), a single examination for assessment of US and international medical school students or graduates seeking initial licensure by US licensing jurisdictions. The USMLE replaced the Federation Licensing Examination (FLEX) and the certification examination of the NBME, as well as the Foreign Medical Graduate Examination in the Medical Sciences (FMGEMS), which was formerly used by the Educational Commission for Foreign Medical Graduates (ECFMG) for certification purposes.

The USMLE is a single examination program with three steps. Each step is complementary to the others; no step can stand alone in the assessment of readiness for medical licensure. For 2010, the fee for the Step 1 examination is $505; Step 2 Clinical Knowledge (CK) is $505 and Step 2 Clinical Skills (CS) is $1,075. Additional information on the USMLE appears on page 90.

Twenty-eight boards do not place any limits on the number of times a candidate for licensure may take USMLE Step 1; similarly, 27 boards do not place limits on taking Step 2. Twenty boards do not limit the amount of time in which a candidate for licensure must pass Steps 1 or 2; most of the boards with such time limits have specified a 7-year time period (Table 1).

Additional Notes for Specific Licensing Jurisdictions

Texas—All candidates, except MD/PhD graduates, must pass all examination steps within 7 years. MD/PhD graduates must pass all steps within 2 years of completing the graduate medical education (GME) required for licensure in Texas. Both of these time limits may be expanded to 10 years if the applicant 1) is specialty board certified by the American Board of Medical Specialties (ABMS) or American Osteopathic Association (AOA) Bureau of Osteopathic Specialists, or 2) has been issued a faculty temporary license in Texas, has practiced under that permit for at least 12 months, and has been recommended for licensure by the institution at which the faculty temporary license was used.

West Virginia—Must appear before licensure committee after 3 failed attempts on any step of the USMLE.

Administration of the United States Medical Licensing Examination Step 3

(See the first two paragraphs on page 2 for general information on the USMLE.)

Many states require US or Canadian medical school graduates to have from 6 to 12 months of accredited US or Canadian GME to take USMLE Step 3. In some states, graduates of foreign medical schools are required to have completed more GME (as much as 3 years in several states). A number of states do not require completion of GME to take Step 3 or require only that a physician taking the examination be enrolled in a GME program (Table 2).

Nearly all medical licensing authorities require completion of Steps 1, 2, and 3 within a 7-year period, or 10 years for those in MD/PhD or similar dual-degree programs (although 21 states may make exceptions in the event of extenuating circumstances, as noted in Table 3). The 7-year period begins when the medical student or graduate first passes Step 1 or Step 2. Thirteen states allow 10 years for completion of all three steps, and eight states do not impose a time limit for completion. Many states limit the number of attempts allowed to pass each step (particularly Step 3) and require additional education, training, or experience after a given number of failed attempts.

For 2010, the fee for the Step 3 examination is $705. Additional information on the USMLE appears on page 90.

Additional Notes for Specific Licensing Jurisdictions

Alabama—If an applicant fails to achieve a passing score on Step 3 in three administrations, the Board may approve one additional attempt to pass Step 3 after *demonstration by the applicant of additional education, experience, or training acceptable to the Board.*

Applicants who are "dual degree candidates" (see definition, below) must achieve a passing score on Step 3 in not more than three administrations and complete Steps 1, 2, and 3 within a 10-year period, beginning when the applicant initially passes his or her first step. The Board does not accept scores from a retaking of a previously passed step of the USMLE.

For purposes of the USMLE, dual degree candidates are defined as the following:

- The applicant is pursuing the MD or DO degree and the PhD degree in an institution or program accredited by the LCME and a regional university accrediting body; and

- The applicant is a student in good standing, enrolled in the institution or program; and

- The PhD studies are in a field of biological sciences tested in the USMLE Step 1 content, including, but not limited to, anatomy, biochemistry, physiology, microbiology, pharmacology, pathology, genetics, neuroscience, and molecular biology.

Arizona—No time limit for USMLE Step 3 for applicants who hold a license in another jurisdiction (licensure by endorsement); for initial licensure, the 7-year limit applies.

Ohio—The applicant shall have passed all three steps within a 10-year period and achieved a recognized passing performance by the USMLE program on each step. No applicant shall have failed any step more than three times.

Any applicant having failed a step more than three times shall do the following to be eligible for licensure:
1) Successfully complete an additional year of GME in addition to that required for licensure. Such education shall be completed subsequent to the final step that has been failed more than three times; and 2) Retake the testing sequence.

Any applicant who has not completed the required steps within the 10-year time period, and has not failed any step more than three times, shall 1) Retake the appropriate steps to bring the testing sequence within the required 10-year time period; or 2) Demonstrate good cause, as determined by the board, for not having passed all three steps within the 10-year period.

Oregon—A waiver is allowed of the three attempt limit for USMLE Step 3 (1 year approved GME after third failed attempt before fourth and final attempt) for applicants who are ABMS certified.

A waiver of the 7-year time limit for completion of USMLE Steps 1, 2, and 3 is allowed for applicants who are ABMS certified, have participated in a combined MD/PhD or DO/PhD program, suffered from a documented significant health condition that by its severity would necessarily cause delay to an applicant's medical study, or have completed continuous GME equivalent to an MD/PhD or DO/PhD program.

Texas—All candidates, except MD/PhD graduates, must pass all examination steps within 7 years. MD/PhD graduates must pass all steps within 2 years of completing the GME required for licensure in Texas. Both of these time limits may be expanded to 10 years if the applicant 1) is ABMS or AOA Bureau of Osteopathic Specialists specialty board certified, or 2) has been issued a faculty temporary license in Texas, has practiced under that permit for at least 12 months, and has been recommended for licensure by the institution at which the faculty temporary license was used.

In addition, although any of the three steps must be passed within three attempts, a fourth attempt is allowed on one step only, and a fifth or sixth attempt is allowed on one step only, if the applicant becomes ABMS or AOA board-certified and completes, in Texas, an additional 2 years of GME beyond what is required.

Virgin Islands—The USMLE is not administered; SPEX is used to evaluate physicians' knowledge.

Washington—All applicants who graduated from medical school after 1993, whether within the US or internationally, are required to pass the USMLE to qualify for licensure.

West Virginia—Must appear before licensure committee after 3 failed attempts on any step of the USMLE.

Table 1
Administration of the US Medical Licensing Examination Steps 1 and 2

	Number of Times Candidates for Licensure May Take USMLE Step 1	Number of Times Candidates for Licensure May Take USMLE Step 2	Amount of Time Within Which Steps 1 and 2 of USMLE Must Be Passed
Alabama	No limit	No limit	No limit
Alaska	2	2	7 yrs
Arizona	No limit	No limit	No limit
Arkansas	6	6	7 yrs
California	No limit	No limit	No limit
Colorado	No limit	No limit	7 yrs (all 3 steps)
Connecticut	No limit	No limit	No limit
Delaware	No limit	No limit	No limit
DC	No limit	No limit	No limit
Florida	No limit	No limit	No limit
Georgia	No limit	No limit	7 yrs (all 3 steps); 9 yrs for MD/PhDs
Guam	Not applicable	Not applicable	Not applicable
Hawaii	No limit	No limit	No limit
Idaho	2	2	7 yrs (all 3 steps)
Illinois	5	5	7 yrs (all 3 steps)
Indiana	3	3	10 yrs (all 3 steps)
Iowa	6	6	10 yrs (all 3 steps)
Kansas	No limit	No limit	10 yrs (all 3 steps)
Kentucky	4	4	No limit
Louisiana	No limit	4	No limit
Maine	No limit	No limit	7 yrs (all 3 steps)
Maryland	4	4	10 yrs (all 3 steps)
Massachusetts	No limit	No limit	7 yrs (all 3 steps)
Michigan	No limit	No limit	No limit
Minnesota	3	3	Before end of training (Step 2)
Mississippi	No limit	No limit	No limit
Missouri	3	3	7 yrs (all 3 steps)
Montana	No limit	No limit	7 yrs (all 3 steps)
Nebraska	4	4	10 yrs (all 3 steps)
Nevada	No limit	No limit	7 yrs (all 3 steps and 9 total attempts) (10 yrs for MD/PhD programs)
New Hampshire	3	3	No limit
New Jersey	No limit	No limit	7 yrs
New Mexico	6	6	7 yrs (all 3 steps)
New York	No limit	No limit	No limit
North Carolina	6	6	7 yrs (all 3 steps); 10 yrs for MD/PhDs
North Dakota	3	3	7 yrs (all 3 steps)

(continued on next page)

Table 1 (continued)
Administration of the US Medical Licensing Examination Steps 1 and 2

	Number of Times Candidates for Licensure May Take USMLE Step 1	Number of Times Candidates for Licensure May Take USMLE Step 2	Amount of Time Within Which Steps 1 and 2 of USMLE Must Be Passed
Ohio	4	4	10 yrs (all 3 steps); no more than 3 failures of any step
Oklahoma	3	3	10 yrs (all 3 steps)
Oregon	No limit	No limit	7 yrs (all 3 steps)
Pennsylvania	No limit	No limit	No limit
Puerto Rico	No limit	No limit	7 yrs
Rhode Island	3	3	7 yrs
South Carolina	3	3	10 yrs (all 3 steps)
South Dakota	3	3	7 yrs (all 3 steps)
Tennessee	No limit	No limit	No limit
Texas*	3	3	7 yrs (all 3 steps); 10 yrs for MD/PhDs
Utah	3	3	7 yrs (10 yrs for MD/PhD programs)
Vermont	No limit	No limit	No limit
Virgin Islands	Not applicable	Not applicable	Not applicable
Virginia	No limit	No limit	No limit
Washington	No limit	No limit	No limit
West Virginia*	3	3	10 yrs
Wisconsin	3	3	10 yrs (all 3 steps)
Wyoming	No limit	No limit	No limit (subject to Board discretion)

* Refer to introductory text to this table for more information on this state's regulations.

Note: All information should be verified with the licensing board; licenses based on endorsement are granted to those physicians meeting all state requirements.

Table 2
Administration of the US Medical Licensing Examination Step 3: Graduate Medical Education Requirements

	Amount of Accredited US or Canadian GME Required to Take USMLE Step 3	
	Graduates of US/Canadian Medical Schools	Graduates of Foreign Medical Schools
Alabama	None (but must be enrolled in GME program)	2 yrs (must be enrolled in third yr of GME program)
Alaska	1 yr	1 yr
Arizona	6 mos	6 mos
Arkansas	None	None
California	None	None
Colorado	1 yr	3 yrs
Connecticut	None	None
Delaware	1 yr	1 yr
DC	1 yr	3 yrs
Florida	None	None
Georgia	1 yr	1-3 yrs
Guam	2 yrs	2 yrs
Hawaii	None (must be enrolled in first yr of GME program)	1 yr (and must be enrolled in second yr of GME program)
Idaho	9 mos	2 yrs, 9 mos
Illinois	1 yr	1 yr
Indiana	1 yr	2 yrs
Iowa	7 mos (or enrollment in approved GME program)	7 mos (or enrollment in approved GME program)
Kansas	1 yr (or enrollment in GME program in Kansas)	3 yrs (2 in US) (or enrollment in GME program in Kansas)
Kentucky	1 yr	1 yr
Louisiana	None	None
Maine	1 yr	1 yr (plus ECFMG certificate)
Maryland	None	None
Massachusetts	1 yr	1 yr
Michigan	6 mos	6 mos
Minnesota	None (but must be enrolled in GME program)	None (but must be enrolled in GME program)
Mississippi	1 yr	1 yr
Missouri	1 yr	3 yrs
Montana	1 yr	1 yr (plus ECFMG)
Nebraska	None	None
Nevada	None	None
New Hampshire	1 yr	1 yr
New Jersey	1 yr	1 yr
New Mexico	1 yr	1 yr
New York	None	None
North Carolina	None	None
North Dakota	6 mos	1 yr
Ohio	9 mos	9 mos
Oklahoma	None	None

(continued on next page)

Table 2 (continued)
Administration of the US Medical Licensing Examination Step 3: Graduate Medical Education Requirements

	Amount of Accredited US or Canadian GME Required to Take USMLE Step 3	
	Graduates of US/Canadian Medical Schools	Graduates of Foreign Medical Schools
Oregon	None (but must be enrolled in GME program)	None (but must be enrolled in GME program)
Pennsylvania	None	None
Puerto Rico	None	None
Rhode Island	1 yr	1 yr
South Carolina	1 yr	3 yrs
South Dakota	None	1 yr
Tennessee	1 yr	1 yr
Texas	None	None
Utah	None	None (must be ECFMG-certified)
Vermont	7 mos	7 mos
Virgin Islands	Not applicable	Not applicable
Virginia	None	None
Washington	1 yr (or enrolled in GME program)	1 yr (or enrolled in GME program)
West Virginia	None	None
Wisconsin	1 yr	1 yr
Wyoming	1 yr	1 yr

Abbreviations

USMLE—United States Medical Licensing Examination
ECFMG—Educational Commission for Foreign Medical Graduates
GME—graduate medical education

Note: *All information should be verified with the licensing board; medical licenses are granted to those physicians meeting all state requirements—at the discretion of the board.*

Table 3
Administration of the US Medical Licensing Examination Step 3: Time Limits for Completion

	Number of Times Candidates for Licensure May Take USMLE Step 3	Requirements to Repeat Step 3 if Not Passed in Designated Number of Attempts	Time Limit for Completion of All Steps of USMLE	Time Limit for MD/PhD or Dual-Degree Candidates	Time Limit May be Waived in Event of Extenuating Circumstances
Alabama*	3	Further education, training, or experience	7 yrs	10 yrs	No
Alaska	2		7 yrs		No
Arizona*	No limit		7 yrs (initial applicants only)		No
Arkansas	6		7 yrs		
California	4 (as of 1/1/07)	—	10 yrs		—
Colorado	No limit		7 yrs	10 yrs	Yes
Connecticut	No limit		7 yrs		No
Delaware	No limit		No limit		No
DC	No limit	After 3 failed attempts, 1 additional yr ACGME- or AOA-approved GME	7 yrs		Yes
Florida	No limit		No limit		—
Georgia	3	1 yr of additional Board-approved training	7 yrs	9 yrs	Yes
Guam	No limit		7 yrs		No
Hawaii	No limit		7 yrs	10 yrs	No
Idaho	2	Remedial training; may be required to be interviewed, evaluated, or examined by the Board	7 yrs	10 yrs	Yes
Illinois	5	Further education, experience, or remedial training	7 yrs		Yes
Indiana	3		10 yrs	10 yrs	No
Iowa	3	After 3 failed attempts, 3 yrs of progressive GME required	10 yrs (If not, ABMS or AOA board certification required)	10 yrs	Yes
Kansas	3	After 3 failed attempts, further education, training, or experience	10 yrs		Yes
Kentucky	4		No limit		No
Louisiana	4		10 yrs		Yes
Maine	3		7 yrs		Yes
Maryland	4	After 3 failed attempts, 1 yr additional GME; no more than 3 failures permitted on any 1 step	10 yrs		No
Massachusetts	6		7 yrs		Yes
Michigan	No limit	After 5 yrs from first attempt, additional GME in Board-approved program in-state	No limit		—
Minnesota	3 (4 if currently licensed in another state and specialty board certified)		Within 5 yrs of passing Step 2 or by end of training		No
Mississippi	3	After 3 failed attempts, 1 additional yr ACGME- or AOA-approved GME	7 yrs		Yes
Missouri	3		7 yrs		No
Montana	3		7 yrs	Exception may be granted	Yes

(continued on next page)

Table 3 (continued)
Administration of the US Medical Licensing Examination Step 3: Time Limits for Completion

	Number of Times Candidates for Licensure May Take USMLE Step 3	Requirements to Repeat Step 3 if Not Passed in Designated Number of Attempts	Time Limit for Completion of All Steps of USMLE	Time Limit for MD/PhD or Dual-Degree Candidates	Time Limit May be Waived in Event of Extenuating Circumstances
Nebraska	4		10 yrs		No
Nevada	3		7 yrs (all 3 steps and 9 total attempts)	10 yrs	Yes (if ABMS certified)
New Hampshire	3	Further education, training, or experience	No limit		—
New Jersey	5	Further education, training, or experience	7 yrs (if not passed, must repeat entire sequence)		Yes
New Mexico	6 (within 7 yrs of first pass)		7 yrs	10 yrs	Yes
New York	No limit		No limit		—
North Carolina	6		7 yrs	10 yrs	Yes
North Dakota	3		7 yrs	Exception may be granted	No
Ohio*	4	Further training; retake entire sequence	10 yrs	10 yrs	Yes
Oklahoma	3		10 yrs	10 yrs	No
Oregon*	4	After 3 failed attempts, 1 yr of GME required before 4th attempt	7 yrs	10 yrs	Yes
Pennsylvania	No limit		No limit		Yes
Puerto Rico	No limit		7 yrs		
Rhode Island	3		7 yrs		Yes
South Carolina	3		10 yrs		No
South Dakota	3		7 yrs	10 yrs	No
Tennessee	No limit		7 yrs		No
Texas*	3		7 yrs	10 yrs	No
Utah	3	Remedial training	7 yrs	10 yrs	No
Vermont	3		7 yrs	10 yrs	No
Virgin Islands*	Not applicable		Not applicable		No
Virginia	No limit		10 yrs		Yes (if ABMS certified)
Washington*	3	Remedial training	7 yrs	10 yrs	Yes
West Virginia*	3	Must appear before licensure committee after 3 failed attempts	10 yrs	10 yrs	No
Wisconsin	3	Must reapply for license and present evidence of further education or training	10 yrs	12 yrs	No
Wyoming	No limit		No limit		

Abbreviations

ABMS—American Board of Medical Specialties
ACGME—Accreditation Council for Graduate Medical Education
AOA—American Osteopathic Association
USMLE—United States Medical Licensing Examination
GME—graduate medical education

* Refer to introductory text to this table for more information on this state's regulations.

Note: All information should be verified with the licensing board; medical licenses are granted to those physicians meeting all state requirements—at the discretion of the board.

Endorsement Policies for Physicians Holding an Initial License

Endorsement is the process through which a state issues an unrestricted license to practice medicine to an individual who holds a valid and unrestricted license in another jurisdiction. Licensure endorsement, previously referred to as "reciprocity," is generally based on documentation of successfully completing approved examinations, authentication of required core documents, and completion of any additional requirements assessing the applicant's fitness to practice medicine in the new jurisdiction. Each state has strict endorsement requirements.

Policies of state licensing boards for endorsement of medical/osteopathic licensing examinations taken before and after the development of the Federation Licensing Examination (FLEX) vary from state to state (Table 4). Each state board created its own licensing examination before FLEX, which may partially explain the sizable variation in endorsement policies from one state to another. Some boards will endorse scores on state licensing examinations in use prior to the development of FLEX; these scores may be endorsed in connection with a passing score on the Special Purpose Examination (SPEX). Endorsement of a certificate of the National Board of Medical Examiners (NBME) or of an examination refers to issuance of a license based on an acceptable score on the NBME or the state's board exam.

Forty-five state medical boards require some or all candidates for licensure endorsement to appear for an interview; three boards require some or all candidates to appear for an oral examination.

Twelve boards require that a license be endorsed within a certain period after examination (usually 10 years). In most of these 12 states, SPEX is required if the time limit is not met.

All medical boards will accept or consider for endorsement the national board certificate of the NBME or the United States Medical Licensing Examination (USMLE), except Texas and the Virgin Islands, which do not accept endorsements. A number of osteopathic boards do not accept USMLE for licensure by endorsement.

Forty-seven boards will endorse the Licentiate of the Medical Council of Canada (LMCC); 37 will endorse the certificates of the National Board of Osteopathic Medical Examiners (NBOME); 31 may endorse a state board examination (designated "SBE" in Table 4) from another jurisdiction, with certain time limitations, and occasionally in combination with a certificate from an American Board of Medical Specialties (ABMS) specialty board; 12 will endorse the Comprehensive Osteopathic Medical Licensing Examination (COMLEX) of the NBOME; seven will endorse FLEX; and two will endorse an ABMS board certificate. (Endorsement of these credentials is subject to any specific requirements in effect in that state.)

Additional Notes for Specific Licensing Jurisdictions

Colorado—LMCC is accepted or considered for endorsement for graduates of US or Canadian medical schools only.

Connecticut—Before June 1985: 75 on day 3 of FLEX to combine best scores (within 7 years); FLEX-Weighted Average (FWA) truncated.

Idaho—FLEX scores obtained at different sittings cannot be combined. Each applicant must pass an examination acceptable to the Board, within the time period recommended by the examination authority, which thoroughly tests the applicant's fitness to practice medicine. If the applicant fails to pass the examination on two separate occasions, the applicant may be required to be interviewed, evaluated, or examined by the Board.

LMCC is endorsed only for graduates of US or Canadian medical schools.

Illinois—Applicant had to pass all three parts of the pre-1985 FLEX in the same state.

Iowa—Applicants who took old (pre-1985) FLEX must provide evidence of at least two of the following: 1) certification under seal that the applicant passed FLEX with a FLEX-weighted average of 75% or better, as determined by the state medical licensing authority, in no more than two sittings; 2) verification under seal of medical licensure in the state that administered the examination; 3) evidence of current certification by an American specialty board approved or recognized by the Council of Medical Education of the AMA or the ABMS or AOA.

Louisiana—At board discretion, candidates for licensure endorsement must appear.

SPEX may be waived if an applicant was certified or recertified by an ABMS board within 10 years of the application date.

Maryland—Licensure by endorsement is not available; the information in Table 4 reflects the requirements for any applicant for initial medical licensure, whether or not another state has issued a license to the applicant.

SPEX is required if an applicant's licensure application was completed more than 15 years ago, the applicant has not maintained uninterrupted licensure in the US, and the applicant has not been certified or recertified by a specialty board within the past 10 years.

Minnesota—SPEX may be waived if the applicant is currently certified by an ABMS board, an AOA specialty board, or a Canadian specialty board.

Mississippi—FLEX scores obtained at different sittings cannot be combined. An exemption may be granted to the weighted average of 75 on FLEX if the applicant has completed an approved GME program and is ABMS or AOA board certified.

LMCC is accepted or considered for endorsement for graduates of US or Canadian medical schools only.

SPEX may be waived if an applicant was certified or recertified by an ABMS board within 10 years of the application date.

North Carolina—Licensure by endorsement requires a valid and unrestricted license to practice medicine in another state based on an examination testing general medical knowledge, or passing of a licensure examination testing general medical knowledge that is determined by the board as equivalent to the board's examination.

Oregon—SPEX may be waived if an applicant was 1) ABMS certified or recertified within 10 years of date of applying for an Oregon license, or 2) completed an accredited 1-year residency or a board-approved clinical fellowship, or 3) obtained CME to the Board's satisfaction.

Texas—Endorsement is not offered. All applicants must meet requirements for initial licensure.

Utah—LMCC is accepted or considered for endorsement for graduates of US or Canadian medical schools only.

Table 4
Endorsement Policies for Physicians Holding an Initial License

	Requirements for Endorsement of License Based on FLEX			Requirements for Candidates' Appearance			Maximum Time for Licensure Endorsement After Examination		Credential Also Accepted or Considered for Endorsement (in Addition to USMLE and NBME)
	Exceptions to 75 FWA on 3-part FLEX	Must Pass 3-Part (Pre-1985) FLEX in One Sitting	Must Pass 2-Part (1985-93) FLEX in One Sitting	Candidates Who Must Appear...	...for Oral Exam	...for Interview	Time	Additional Requirements if Time Limit Not Met	
Alabama	None	No	No	Some			10 yrs	SPEX, ABMS	LMCC
Alaska	None	No	No	Some		X	None		LMCC, NBOME
Arizona	None	Yes	No	Some		X	None		LMCC
Arizona DO	None	No	No	Some	X	X	7 yrs		SBE (pre-FLEX), NBOME
Arkansas	None	Yes	No	IMGs		X	None		LMCC
California	None	Yes	No	None			None		LMCC
California DO	None	No	No	None					NBOME
Colorado*	None	Yes	No	None			None		LMCC
Connecticut*	See note	No	No	None			None		LMCC, SBE, NBOME
Delaware	None	No	No	All		X	None		LMCC
DC	None	Yes	No	None			None		LMCC, NBOME
Florida	None	Yes	No	Some		X	None		
Florida DO	NA	NA	NA	Some		X	None		SBE, NBOME, COMVEX
Georgia	None	Yes	No	Some		X	None		LMCC, NBOME COMLEX
Guam	None	Yes	Yes	Some		X	10 yrs	SPEX	NBOME
Hawaii	None	No	No	None			None		
Hawaii DO	None	No	No	None			None		NBOME
Idaho*	See note	Yes	No	Some		X	5 yrs	SPEX	LMCC, SBE, NBOME
Illinois*	None	No	No	Some		X	None		LMCC, NBOME
Indiana	Split scores okay	No	No	Some		X	None		LMCC
Iowa*	See note	No	No	Some		X	None		LMCC, SBE, NBOME
Kansas	None	Yes	No	Some		X	None		LMCC, SBE (pre-'72) NBOME, COMLEX
Kentucky	None	Yes	No	Some			None		LMCC, NBOME, COMLEX
Louisiana*	None	Yes	No	Some		X	10 yrs	SPEX	SBE
Maine	None	No	No	Some		X	None		LMCC, SBE, GMC
Maine DO	None	No	No	Some		X	None	SPEX	NBOME
Maryland*	None	Yes	No	None			15 yrs	SPEX	LMCC, NBOME, COMLEX
Massachusetts	None	Yes	Yes	Some		X	None	Current evaluations	LMCC, NBOME, COMLEX, SBE (prior to 6/19/70)
Michigan	None	Yes	No	None			None		LMCC, SBE
Michigan DO	NA	NA	NA	None					NBOME, SBE (pre-FLEX)
Minnesota*	None	Yes (5 tries)	No (3 tries)	All		X	10 yrs	SPEX, ABMS	LMCC, SBE, NBOME, COMLEX
Mississippi*	See note	Yes	No	All		X	10 yrs	SPEX, ABMS	LMCC, SBE (pre-1973), NBOME
Missouri	None	Yes	No	Some		X	None		LMCC, NBOME
Montana	None	No	No	Some		X	None		LMCC, NBOME

(continued on next page)

Table 4 (continued)
Endorsement Policies for Physicians Holding an Initial License

	Requirements for Endorsement of License Based on FLEX			Requirements for Candidates' Appearance			Maximum Time for Licensure Endorsement After Examination		Credential Also Accepted or Considered for Endorsement (in Addition to USMLE and NBME)
	Exceptions to 75 FWA on 3-part FLEX	Must Pass 3-Part (Pre-1985) FLEX in One Sitting	Must Pass 2-Part (1985-92) FLEX in One Sitting	Candidates Who Must Appear...	...for Oral Exam	...for Interview	Time	Additional Requirements if Time Limit Not Met	
Nebraska	None	Yes	No	None			None		LMCC, SBE
Nevada	None	No	No	Some		X	None		LMCC
Nevada DO	None	No	No	None			10 yrs	ABMS exam, COMVEX, SPEX	SBE (pre-FLEX) NBOME
New Hampshire	None	No	No	None			None	May require exam, interview, proof of clinical competence, etc	LMCC, SBE
New Jersey	Pre-Jan 1981: 74.5 FWA	No	No	Some		X	None		LMCC w/ABMS & SBE; ABMS w/SBE
New Mexico	None	No	No	Some		X	None		LMCC, SBE, FLEX (pre-1974)
New Mexico DO	None	No	No	All		X			NBOME, FLEX, COMLEX
New York	None	No; 5-yr period to pass all parts	No; 5-yr period to pass all parts	None			None		LMCC (with a valid Canadian provincial license), ABMS, foreign license
North Carolina*	None	No	No	Some		X	10 yrs	Training, SPEX, AMA PRA, ABMS	LMCC, SBE, FLEX, NBOME, COMLEX
North Dakota	None	Yes	No	Some		X	None		LMCC, SBE, NBOME, COMLEX
Ohio	72 if taken during first 2 yrs of a state's administration and accepted as passing by state	Yes	No	None			None		LMCC (professional experience in US or abroad)
Oklahoma	None	Yes	No	Some		X	None		LMCC
Oklahoma DO	NA			Some		X			NBOME
Oregon*	None	Yes	No	Some		X	10 yrs	SPEX	LMCC, NBOME, SBE, FLEX, COMLEX
Pennsylvania	None	No	No	None			None		LMCC
Pennsylvania DO	None	No	No	None			None		SBE, NBOME, FLEX
Puerto Rico	None	Yes	Yes	None			None		
Rhode Island	None	No	No	Some		X	None		LMCC, NBOME
South Carolina	None	Yes	No	All		X	10 yrs	SPEX	LMCC, SBE w/ABMS, NBOME
South Dakota	None	Yes	Yes	Some		X	None		LMCC, NBOME, SBE, FLEX, COMLEX
Tennessee	None	Yes	Yes	Some		X	None		LMCC, ABMS
Tennessee DO	None	No	No	Some		X			NBOME
Texas*	—	—	—	—	—	—	—	—	—
Utah*	None	No	No	Some		X	None	Retake exams	LMCC, SBE
Vermont	None	Yes	Yes	All		X	None		LMCC, SBE, FLEX
Vermont DO	None	No	No	None					SBE (pre-FLEX), NBOME

(continued on next page)

Table 4 (continued)
Endorsement Policies for Physicians Holding an Initial License

	Requirements for Endorsement of License Based on FLEX			Requirements for Candidates' Appearance			Maximum Time for Licensure Endorsement After Examination		Credential Also Accepted or Considered for Endorsement (in Addition to USMLE and NBME)
	Exceptions to 75 FWA on 3-part FLEX	Must Pass 3-Part (Pre-1985) FLEX in One Sitting	Must Pass 2-Part (1985-92) FLEX in One Sitting	Candidates Who Must Appear...	...for Oral Exam	...for Interview	Time	Additional Requirements if Time Limit Not Met	
Virgin Islands	No reciprocity or endorsement; all licensure candidates must sit for complete SPEX exam.								
Virginia	None	No (unless taken pre-June 1976)	Yes	Some		X	None		LMCC, pre-1970=SBE, with ABMS
Washington	None	No	No	None			None		LMCC (post-1969)
Washington DO	None	No	No	None					SBE (pre-FLEX), NBOME
West Virginia	None	Yes	No	All		X	None		LMCC, SBE
West Virginia DO	NA	NA	NA	All		X			SBE (pre-FLEX) NBOME
Wisconsin	None	Yes	No	Some	X	X	None		LMCC (post-1978)
Wyoming	None	Yes	No	Some	X	X	None		LMCC, SBE, NBOME COMLEX

Abbreviations

FWA—Federation Licensing Examination (FLEX) Weighted Average, which applied to the pre-1985 three-part FLEX and gave greater weight to parts 2 and 3; all states currently require a minimum passing score of 75 on each component of the post-1985 two-part FLEX.

ABMS—certification from a member board of the American Board of Medical Specialties

COMLEX—Comprehensive Osteopathic Medical Licensing Examination

COMVEX—Comprehensive Osteopathic Medical Variable-Purpose Examination

FLEX—Federation Licensing Examination

GMC—General Medical Council of the United Kingdom

IMG—international medical graduate

LMCC—certification by the Licentiate of the Medical Council of Canada

NBME—certificate of the National Board of Medical Examiners

NBOME—certificate from the National Board of Osteopathic Medical Examiners

SBE—state board examination

SPEX—Special Purpose Examination

USMLE—United States Medical Licensing Examination

* Refer to introductory text to this table for more information on this state's regulations.

Note: *All information should be verified with the licensing board; licenses based on endorsement are granted to those physicians meeting all state requirements.*

Additional Requirements for Endorsement of Licenses Held by International Medical Graduates (IMGs)

In all states, international medical graduates (IMGs) seeking licensure by endorsement must meet the same requirements as US graduates (listed in Table 4), in addition to the requirements shown in Table 5.

All states except California and West Virginia require that IMGs seeking licensure endorsement hold a certificate from the Educational Commission for Foreign Medical Graduates (ECFMG). In lieu of holding that certificate, a candidate for licensure in North Dakota may have passed a certification examination of an American Board of Medical Specialties (ABMS) board.

About half of the boards require IMG candidates to have graduated from a state-approved foreign medical school; several boards also maintain and use a list of approved/unapproved foreign medical schools for decisions on initial licensure (see Table 9, column 3). A number of boards require 2 or 3 years of US or Canadian GME, and a majority of jurisdictions also may require an interview or oral examination prior to endorsement.

Note: Physicians who graduated via the Fifth Pathway are not required to have an ECFMG certificate. For more information on the Fifth Pathway, see page 28.

Additional Notes for Specific Licensing Jurisdictions

California—Four years' licensure required for IMGs, in addition to 2 years of ACGME-accredited training (or 1 year of ACGME-accredited training plus ABMS, or 1 year of ACGME-accredited training plus SPEX).

Florida—Rules on clinical clerkships for IMGs adopted by the Florida Board before October 1986 do not apply to any graduate who had already completed a clinical clerkship or who had begun a clinical clerkship, as long as the clerkship was completed within 3 years.

Illinois—Candidate must have completed a 6-year postsecondary course of study, comprising 2 academic years of liberal arts instruction, 2 academic years in basic sciences, and 2 academic years in clinical sciences, while enrolled in the medical school that confirmed the degree.

Iowa—Requirement for graduation from a state-approved medical school is waived if candidate passed the Special Purpose Examination (SPEX) or state science examination, or completed 3 years of GME in an ACGME-accredited residency program, or held a permanent license to practice without restrictions in a US jurisdiction for at least 5 years.

Maryland—In addition to 2 years of ACGME- or Royal College of Physicians and Surgeons of Canada (RCPSC)-accredited GME, 1 year of GME required if candidate failed any part of an examination three times; no more than three failures permitted.

Minnesota—SPEX is required if candidate took initial licensing exam more than 10 years ago, unless candidate is currently ABMS/AOA or Canadian medical specialty board certified.

North Dakota—The ECFMG certificate requirement is waived for holders of the Fifth Pathway and for graduates of medical schools in Canada, England, Scotland, Ireland, Australia, or New Zealand. The requirement may be waived, by unanimous vote of the Board, for holders of ABMS certification.

The requirement for 3 years of US/Canadian GME is waived if the candidate holds an ABMS board certificate or has passed SPEX and 1) has successfully completed 1 year of state-approved GME in the US or Canada (or 3 years of GME in the United Kingdom), 2) has other professional experience and training equivalent to GME years 2 and 3, and 3) meets all other licensing requirements.

Oregon—Candidate must have graduated from a foreign school listed that provided instruction equivalent to a US medical school and is considered equivalent if on the list of medical schools recognized by the Medical Board of California or one of the countries listed by the US Department of Education's National Committee on Foreign Medical Education and Accreditation (NCFMEA). Medical school must be chartered in country in which it is located; candidate must attend four full terms of 8 months each term, with physical on-site attendance. The four full terms of 8 months each term may be waived for candidates with ABMS certificates who have substantially complied with attendance requirements.

Rhode Island—Candidate must have obtained supervised clinical training in the US as part of the medical school curriculum in a hospital affiliated with an LCME-accredited medical school or an ACGME-accredited residency.

Table 5
Additional Requirements for Endorsement of Licenses Held by International Medical Graduates (IMGs)
IMGs must also meet all the requirements for endorsement listed in Table 4

	Must Have ECFMG Certificate	Must Have Graduated From State-approved Foreign Medical School (cf Table 9, Column 3)	Must Appear for...		Amount of Accredited US or Canadian GME Required	Notes
			Interview	Possible Interview		
Alabama	Yes	Yes				SPEX (if no ABMS or SBE within 10 yrs)
Alaska	Yes	Yes		Yes		
Arizona	Yes	No			3 yrs	
Arkansas	Yes	Yes	Yes		3 yrs	
California*	No	Yes				
Colorado	Yes	Yes			3 yrs	Foreign med school must be board-approved, on case-by-case basis, if applicant is not board certified
Connecticut	Yes	Yes				Foreign med school must have been listed with the World Health Organization in 1970 (or by individual review)
Delaware	Yes	No	Yes			
DC	Yes	No				
Florida*	Yes	No		Yes	2 yrs	
Georgia	Yes	Yes		Yes	3 yrs	1 yr if graduated from medical school before 7/1/1985
Guam	Yes	No		Yes		
Hawaii	Yes	No			2 yrs	
Idaho	Yes	Yes		Yes	3 yrs	Unapproved medical school graduates must meet additional requirements
Illinois*	Yes	No		Yes	2 yrs	
Indiana	Yes	Yes		Yes	2 yrs	
Iowa*	Yes	Yes		Yes	2 yrs	2 yrs of US/Canadian GME required as of 7/1/06
Kansas	Yes	No		Yes	2 yrs	Foreign med school must have been in existence 15 yrs
Kentucky	Yes	Yes		Yes	2 yrs	
Louisiana	Yes	Yes	Yes		3 yrs	
Maine	Yes	Yes		Yes	3 yrs	Foreign medical school must be listed with ECFMG
Maryland*	Yes	No			2 yrs	
Massachusetts	Yes	No		Yes	2 yrs	
Michigan	Yes	No			2 yrs	
Minnesota*	Yes	Yes	Yes		2 yrs	SPEX is required
Mississippi	Yes	Yes	Yes		3 yrs	1 yr if ABMS- or AOA-certified
Missouri	Yes	Yes		Yes	3 yrs	
Montana	Yes	Yes		Yes	3 yrs	
Nebraska	Yes	No			3 yrs	
Nevada	Yes	Yes		Yes	3 yrs	SPEX (if no ABMS or NBME/FLEX/USMLE within 10 yrs)
New Hampshire	Yes	No			2 yrs	
New Jersey	Yes	No		Yes		
New Mexico	Yes	Yes		Yes		Must be board certified in ABMS-recognized specialty and have practiced for past 3 yrs in US/Canada
New York	Yes	No				
North Carolina	Yes	No		Yes	3 yrs	

(continued on next page)

Table 5 (continued)
Additional Requirements for Endorsement of Licenses Held by International Medical Graduates (IMGs)
IMGs must also meet all the requirements for endorsement listed in Table 4

| | Must Have ECFMG Certificate | Must Have Graduated From State-approved Foreign Medical School (cf Table 9, Column 3) | Must Appear for... | | Amount of Accredited US or Canadian GME Required | Notes |
			Interview	Possible Interview		
North Dakota*	Yes	Yes		Yes	3 yrs	
Ohio	Yes	No			2 yrs	
Oklahoma	Yes	Yes			2 yrs	
Oregon*	Yes	Yes		Yes	3 yrs	
Pennsylvania	Yes	No		Yes	3 yrs	Foreign medical school must be listed with ECFMG
Puerto Rico	Yes	Yes				
Rhode Island*	Yes	Yes		Yes	3 yrs	1 yr of advanced standing recognized if granted by ABMS
South Carolina	Yes	No	Yes		3 yrs	For Fifth Pathway candidates, ABMS/AOA cert. required
South Dakota	Yes	Yes		Yes	3 yrs	Must complete a residency program
Tennessee	Yes	Yes		Yes		
Texas*	—	—	—	—	—	Endorsement is not offered. All applicants must meet requirements for initial licensure.
Utah	Yes	No		Yes	2 yrs	
Vermont	Yes	Yes	Yes		3 yrs	
Virginia	Yes	No		Yes	2 yrs	Licensure in another state can replace ECFMG cert.
Washington	Yes	No			2 yrs	
West Virginia	No	No	Yes		3 yrs	3 yrs GME, or 1 yr plus ABMS certification
Wisconsin	Yes	No			1 yr	Possible oral exam
Wyoming	Yes	No			2 yrs	

Abbreviations

ABMS—American Board of Medical Specialties

AOA—American Osteopathic Association

ECFMG—Educational Commission for Foreign Medical Graduates

FLEX—Federation Licensing Examination

FMGEMS—Foreign Medical Graduate Examination in the Medical Sciences

GME—Graduate medical education

IMG—international medical graduate

NBME—National Board of Medical Examiners

SBE—state board examination

SPEX—Special Purpose Examination

USMLE—United States Medical Licensing Examination

VQE—Visa Qualifying Examination

* Refer to introductory text to this table for more information on this state's regulations.

Note: *All information should be verified with the licensing board; licenses based on endorsement are granted to those physicians meeting all state requirements.*

Policies About the Special Purpose Examination (SPEX) and Comprehensive Osteopathic Medical Variable-Purpose Examination (COMVEX)

The Special Purpose Examination (SPEX), a 1-day, computer-administered examination with approximately 420 multiple-choice questions, assesses knowledge required of all physicians, regardless of specialty. SPEX is used to assess physicians who have held a valid, unrestricted license in a US or Canadian jurisdiction who are:

- Required by the state medical board to demonstrate current medical knowledge
- Seeking endorsement licensure some years beyond initial examination
- Seeking license reinstatement after a period of professional inactivity

Physicians holding a valid, unrestricted license may also apply for SPEX, independent of any request or approval from a medical licensing board.

For more information on SPEX, see page 98.

The Comprehensive Osteopathic Medical Variable-Purpose Examination (COMVEX-USA) is a post-licensure examination for osteopathic physicians who require reevaluation after initial licensure. The examination contains 400 test items using objective type questions such as multiple choice, single best answer, and matching test items.

COMVEX may be used in a number of situations, including but not limited to the following:

- An osteopathic physician originally licensed through an examination devoid of osteopathic content is now applying for a license in a state that requires that an osteopathic physician take an osteopathic examination
- An osteopathic physician is applying for licensure in a state that imposes a time limit (e.g., completing examination within a 10-year period), and the candidate has not been tested by a licensing board or a certifying board within that time frame
- An osteopathic physician is requesting a reinstatement of a license following a career interruption
- A tenured osteopathic physician needs to demonstrate basic osteopathic medical competence

For more information on COMVEX, see page 102.

Fifty-nine jurisdictions use SPEX or COMVEX to assess current competence or if a candidate has not taken a written licensure exam or the American Board of Medical Specialties (ABMS) board certification examination within a specified number of years (usually 10). In 27 jurisdictions, SPEX or COMVEX scores are valid for an unlimited length of time. Forty-four jurisdictions will accept SPEX scores from other licensing jurisdictions (Table 6).

For more information on physician reentry to practice, see Table 20.

Additional Notes for Specific Licensing Jurisdictions

Florida—SPEX is offered only to candidates who have actively practiced medicine for at least 10 years after obtaining a valid license in a jurisdiction or a combination of jurisdictions in the United States or Canada and who meet Florida's licensure requirements.

Maryland—SPEX is required if active licensure was interrupted during the last 10 years and if a physician has not passed a written licensure examination within the last 15 years and an ABMS board certification examination within the last 10 years.

North Dakota—SPEX (or ABMS board certification) is required when a candidate is being considered for the following exception: If the candidate has not completed 3 years of GME but has met all other licensing requirements and has successfully completed 1 year of US or Canadian GME in a board-approved program, and if the board finds that the candidate has other professional experience and training substantially equivalent to the second and third years of GME, then the candidate may be eligible for licensure.

Texas—SPEX scores accepted from other licensing jurisdictions if a candidate passed with a score of 75 or higher.

Vermont DO—SPEX or COMVEX, or both, may be required to reinstate an expired license.

West Virginia DO—COMVEX may be required.

Table 6
Policies About the Special Purpose Examination (SPEX) and Comprehensive Osteopathic Medical Variable-Purpose Examination (COMVEX)

	SPEX or COMVEX May Be Required...	...for the Following Reasons	...to Assess Current Competence	...if Written Licensure Exam or Board Certification Exam Has Not Been Taken Within	SPEX/COMVEX Scores Valid for	SPEX/COMVEX Scores Accepted From Other Jurisdictions
Alabama	Yes	By board order	X	10 yrs	10 yrs	Yes
Alaska	Yes	To restore a retired license	X		No limit	Optional
Arizona	Yes	By board order	X		10 yrs	Yes
Arizona DO	Yes	By board order	X	7 yrs		
Arkansas	Yes	By board order	X			Yes
California	Yes		X	10 yrs	10 yrs	Yes
California DO	Yes	By board order	X			No
Colorado	Yes	By board order	X			Yes
Connecticut	Yes		X			Yes
Delaware	No					
DC	Yes	By board order	X			No
Florida*	Yes		X		No limit	Yes
Florida DO	Yes	By board order, or 2 NBOME steps taken				
Georgia	Yes	By board order	X			Yes
Guam	Yes	By board order	X	10 yrs	No limit	Yes
Hawaii	Yes	If MD took a state licensing exam			No limit	Yes
Hawaii DO	No					
Idaho	Yes	By board order	X		No limit	Yes
Illinois	Yes	Restore license after disciplinary action; if not been practicing for several yrs	X		No limit	Yes
Indiana	Yes	If not been practicing; by board order	X		No limit	Yes
Iowa	Yes	If not practicing for several yrs	X		No limit	Yes
Kansas	Yes	By board order	X		No limit	Yes
Kentucky	Yes	By board order	X		No limit	No
Louisiana	Yes		X	10 yrs	10 yrs	Yes
Maine	Yes	If not practicing for > 1 yr	X		No limit	No
Maine DO	Yes	If not practicing for > 1 yr or by board order	X		No limit	No
Maryland*	Yes	If no active licensure in the US within last 10 yrs	X	15 yrs (licensure exam) 10 yrs (ABMS exam)	No limit	Yes
Massachusetts	No					No
Michigan	Yes	By board order	X			Yes
Michigan DO	Yes	By board order	X			Yes
Minnesota	Yes	Restore license after disciplinary action	X	10 yrs	No limit (3 attempts)	Yes
Mississippi	Yes	Restore license after disciplinary action	X	10 yrs	10 yrs	Yes
Missouri	Yes	Restore license after disciplinary action	X		No limit	Yes
Montana	Yes	If not practicing or inactive Montana license for last 2 yrs	X		No limit	Yes
Nebraska	Yes		X			Yes
Nevada	Yes	To meet the 10-yr exam rule or to prove clinical competency	X	10 yrs	10 yrs	Yes

(continued on next page)

Table 6 (continued)
Policies About the Special Purpose Examination (SPEX) and Comprehensive Osteopathic Medical Variable-Purpose Examination (COMVEX)

	SPEX or COMVEX May Be Required...	...for the Following Reasons	...to Assess Current Competence	...if Written Licensure Exam or Board Certification Exam Has Not Been Taken Within	SPEX/COMVEX Scores Valid for	SPEX/COMVEX Scores Accepted From Other Jurisdictions
Nevada DO	Yes	By board order	X	10 yrs	10 yrs	Yes
New Hampshire	Yes	By board order				No
New Jersey	No					No
New Mexico	Yes	Restore license after disciplinary action; if not practicing for several yrs	X		Not defined	Yes
New Mexico DO	Yes	Determined on individual basis				
New York	Yes	Determined on individual basis	X	(If state board exam taken before 1968)	No limit	Yes
North Carolina	Yes	Determined on individual basis	X	10 yrs	10 yrs	Yes
North Dakota*	Yes	(See note)	X		No limit	Yes
Ohio	Yes	If not practicing for 2 yrs	X		No limit	Yes
Oklahoma	Yes	Determined on individual basis	X			Yes
Oklahoma DO	Yes		X			
Oregon	Yes	If not practicing for 1 yr, or no training or ABMS cert. for 10 yrs	X	10 yrs (or if state board exam taken before 1968)	10 yrs	Yes
Pennsylvania	Yes	Restore license after disciplinary action; if not practicing for several yrs	X			Yes
Pennsylvania DO	Yes	Restore license after disciplinary action	X			Yes
Puerto Rico	No					Yes
Rhode Island	No					No
South Carolina	Yes	Restore license after disciplinary action	X	10 yrs	10 yrs	No
South Dakota	No					No
Tennessee	Yes	Restore license after disciplinary action; if license retired > 5 yrs	X		No limit	Yes
Tennessee DO	No					
Texas*	Yes		X	10 yrs	10 yrs	Yes
Utah	Yes	If not practicing for several yrs; restore license after discipline	X	10 yrs (DOs only)	Not defined	Yes
Vermont	No					No
Vermont DO*	Yes	Restore license if not practicing for >1 yr				
Virgin Islands	Yes	To obtain licensure	X		No limit	No
Virginia	Yes		X		No limit	No
Washington	Yes	Restore license after disciplinary action; if not practicing for 2+ yrs or on a case-by-case basis	X		No limit	Yes
Washington DO	Yes	If not practicing for 3 yrs	X		No limit	No
West Virginia*	Yes		X		No limit	Yes
West Virginia DO	Yes		X			Yes
Wisconsin	Yes	Determined on individual basis	X		No limit	Yes
Wyoming	Yes	Determined on individual basis	X		No limit	Yes

Abbreviations

ABMS—American Board of Medical Specialties

COMVEX—Comprehensive Osteopathic Medical Variable-Purpose Examination

SPEX—Special Purpose Examination

* Refer to introductory text to this table for more on this state's regulations.

Note: *All information should be verified with the licensing board; medical licenses are granted to those physicians meeting all state requirements—at the discretion of the board.*

Initial Licensure of US Medical/ Osteopathic School Graduates

All states require a written examination for initial licensure: generally, for MDs, the three-step United States Medical Licensing Examination (USMLE), which has replaced the Federation Licensing Examination (FLEX) and the national board examination of the National Board of Medical Examiners (NBME). Osteopathic physicians take the three-level Comprehensive Osteopathic Medical Licensing Examination (COMLEX-USA) of the National Board of Osteopathic Medical Examiners (NBOME).

To be eligible to take USMLE Step 3, more than half of the state medical boards require graduates of US medical schools to have completed at least 1 year of graduate medical education (GME) (Table 7). Twenty-four boards do not require completion of any GME to take USMLE Step 3 (although in some cases a candidate must be enrolled in a GME program).

To be eligible to take Level 3 of the Comprehensive Osteopathic Medical Licensing Examination (COMLEX), osteopathic physicians must be currently participating in and in good standing with an AOA-accredited internship or ACGME-accredited GME program or must have successfully completed such an internship or program.

All medical and osteopathic boards require completion of at least 1 year of GME before issuing a full, unrestricted license.

Table 7
Initial Licensure of US Medical/Osteopathic School Graduates

	Amount of Accredited US or Canadian GME Required	
	...to Take USMLE Step 3 or COMLEX Level 3	...for Licensure
Alabama	None (must be enrolled in GME program)	1 yr
Alaska	1 yr	2 yrs (1 yr if completed medical school before Jan. 1995)
Arizona	6 mos	1 yr
Arizona DO	6 mos of a 1-yr AOA- or ACGME-accredited program	1 yr AOA- or ACGME-accredited GME
Arkansas	None	1 yr
California	None	1 yr (including 4 mos general medicine)
California DO	1-yr AOA- or ACGME-accredited program	1 yr AOA- or ACGME-accredited GME, including at least 4 mos general medicine (unless applicant completed 1 yr of GME before July 1, 1990).
Colorado	1 yr	1 yr
Connecticut	None	2 yrs
Delaware	1 yr	1 yr
DC	1 yr	1 yr
Florida	None	1 yr
Florida DO	6 mos of a 1-yr AOA- or ACGME-accredited program	1 yr AOA-approved rotating internship
Georgia	1 yr	1 yr
Guam	2 yrs	
Hawaii	None (must be enrolled in 1st yr of GME prgm)	1 yr
Hawaii DO	None	1 yr AOA- or ACGME-accredited GME
Idaho	9 mos	1 yr
Illinois	1 yr	2 yrs (1 yr if entered GME before Jan. 1988)
Indiana	1 yr (6 mos may be waived)	1 yr
Iowa	7 mos (or enrollment in board-approved program)	1 yr AOA-, ACGME-, RCPSC-, CFPC-accredited GME
Kansas	1 yr (or enrollment in GME program in Kansas)	1 yr
Kentucky	1 yr	2 yrs
Louisiana	None	1 yr allopathic GME
Maine	1 yr	3 yrs (for those graduating after 7/1/2004)
Maine DO	1-yr AOA- or ACGME-accredited program	1 yr AOA- or ACGME-accredited GME
Maryland	None (1 yr if 3 fails on any Step)	1 yr (plus 1 yr GME if candidate failed any part of an exam 3 times)
Massachusetts	1 yr	1 yr
Michigan	6 mos	2 yrs
Michigan DO	None	1 yr AOA-approved GME
Minnesota	None (must be enrolled in GME program)	1 yr
Mississippi	1 yr	1 yr
Missouri	1 yr	1 yr
Montana	1 yr	2 yrs
Nebraska	None	1 yr
Nevada	None	3 yrs
Nevada DO	6 mos of a 1-yr AOA- or ACGME-accredited program	3 yrs in AOA- or ACGME-accredited program (grads after 1995)

(continued on next page)

Table 7 (continued)
Initial Licensure of US Medical/Osteopathic School Graduates

	Amount of Accredited US or Canadian GME Required	
	...to Take USMLE Step 3 or COMLEX Level 3	...for Licensure
New Hampshire	1 yr	2 yrs
New Jersey	1 yr	2 yrs, and contract for yr 3, if graduated after July 1, 2003; 1 yr if graduated before July 1, 2003
New Mexico	1 yr	2 yrs
New Mexico DO	6 mos of a 1-yr AOA- or ACGME-accredited program	1 yr
New York	None	1 yr
North Carolina	None	1 yr
North Dakota	6 mos of a 1-yr ACGME- or AOA-accredited program	1 yr
Ohio	9 mos	1 yr
Oklahoma	None	1 yr
Oklahoma DO	6 mos of a 1-yr AOA- or ACGME-accredited program	1 yr AOA-approved rotating internship or equivalent
Oregon	None (must be enrolled in GME program)	1 yr
Pennsylvania	None	2 yrs (1 yr if GME in US before July 1987)
Pennsylvania DO	6 mos of a 1-yr AOA- or ACGME-accredited program	1 yr AOA-approved rotating internship
Puerto Rico	None	1 yr
Rhode Island	1 yr	2 yrs
South Carolina	1 yr	1 yr
South Dakota	None	Completion of residency program
Tennessee	1 yr	1 yr
Tennessee DO	6 mos of a 1-yr AOA- or ACGME-accredited program	1-yr AOA-approved or ACGME-accredited GME
Texas	None	1 yr
Utah	None	2 yrs
Vermont	7 mos	1 yr (Canadian GME accepted if program accredited by RCPSC or CFPC)
Vermont DO	6 mos of a 1-yr AOA- or ACGME-accredited program	1 yr AOA-approved rotating internship or 3-yr AOA- or ACGME-accredited GME program
Virgin Islands	USMLE not offered	1 yr
Virginia	None	1 yr
Washington	1 yr (or enrolled in GME program)	2 yrs (1 yr if completed medical school before July 28, 1985)
Washington DO	6 mos of a 1-yr AOA- or ACGME-accredited program	1 yr AOA-approved or ACGME-accredited GME
West Virginia	None	1 yr
West Virginia DO	6 mos of a 1-yr AOA- or ACGME-accredited program	1 yr AOA-approved or ACGME-accredited GME
Wisconsin	1 yr	1 yr
Wyoming	1 yr	1 yr

Abbreviations

ACGME—Accreditation Council for Graduate Medical Education

AOA—American Osteopathic Association

CFPC—College of Family Physicians of Canada

COMLEX—Comprehensive Osteopathic Medical Licensing Examination

GME—graduate medical education

RCPSC—Royal College of Physicians and Surgeons of Canada

USMLE—United States Medical Licensing Examination

Note: *All information should be verified with the licensing board; medical licenses are granted to those physicians meeting all state requirements—at the discretion of the board.*

Initial Licensure of Canadian Citizens Who Are Graduates of Accredited Canadian Medical Schools

When considering applications for licensure, all state medical boards consider Canadian citizens who have graduated from an accredited Canadian medical school on the same basis as graduates of accredited US medical schools (Table 8).

Forty-six licensing boards endorse the Licentiate of the Medical Council of Canada (LMCC) as evidence of passing an acceptable licensing examination (applicants must also pass all other board requirements for licensure).

With the exception of Guam and the Virgin Islands, all licensing boards accept Canadian graduate medical education (GME) as equivalent to GME in a US program accredited by the Accreditation Council for Graduate Medical Education (ACGME). These rules do not uniformly apply to international medical graduates, who should refer to Table 9.

Table 8
Initial Licensure of Canadian Citizens Who Are Graduates of Accredited Canadian Medical Schools

	LMCC Approved for Licensure by Endorsement	GME in Accredited Canadian Programs Accepted as Equivalent to ACGME-accredited GME in the United States	Notes
Alabama	Yes	Yes	
Alaska	Yes	Yes	
Arizona	Yes	Yes	
Arkansas	Yes	Yes	
California	Yes	Yes	
Colorado	Yes	Yes	
Connecticut	Yes	Yes	
Delaware	Yes	Yes	
DC	Yes	Yes	
Florida	No	Yes	
Georgia	Yes	Yes	
Guam	No	No	
Hawaii	No	Yes	
Idaho	Yes	Yes	
Illinois	Yes	Yes	
Indiana	Yes	Yes	
Iowa	Yes	Yes	LMCC must be endorsed by provincial licensing board
Kansas	Yes	Yes	
Kentucky	Yes	Yes	
Louisiana	No	Yes	
Maine	Yes	Yes	LMCC, subject to board approval
Maryland	Yes	Yes	LMCC (although applicants are not licensed by endorsement)
Massachusetts	Yes	Yes	
Michigan	Yes	Yes	
Minnesota	Yes	Yes	
Mississippi	Yes	Yes	
Missouri	Yes	Yes	Only if medical school graduate of Canadian medical school
Montana	Yes	Yes	
Nebraska	Yes	Yes	
Nevada	Yes	Yes	
New Hampshire	Yes	Yes	
New Jersey	No	Yes	LMCC considered *only* if applicant is licensed in US jurisdiction
New Mexico	Yes	Yes	
New York	Yes	Yes	LMCC considered *only* if applicant has valid provincial license
North Carolina	Yes	Yes	
North Dakota	Yes	Yes	
Ohio	Yes	Yes	1 yr of GME or its equivalent required

(continued on next page)

Table 8 (continued)
Initial Licensure of Canadian Citizens Who Are Graduates of Accredited Canadian Medical Schools

	LMCC Approved for Licensure by Endorsement	GME in Accredited Canadian Programs Accepted as Equivalent to ACGME-accredited GME in the United States	Notes
Oklahoma	Yes	Yes	
Oregon	Yes	Yes	
Pennsylvania	Yes	Yes	Must have received LMCC after 5/70 and in English
Puerto Rico	No	Yes	LMCC considered *only* if applicant is licensed in US jurisdiction
Rhode Island	Yes	Yes	
South Carolina	Yes	Yes	
South Dakota	Yes	Yes	
Tennessee	Yes	Yes	
Texas	—	Yes	Endorsement is not offered. All applicants must meet requirements for initial licensure.
Utah	Yes	Yes	
Vermont	Yes	Yes	
Virgin Islands	No	No	
Virginia	Yes	Yes	
Washington	Yes	Yes	Must have received LMCC after 12/69
West Virginia	Yes	Yes	
Wisconsin	Yes	Yes	Must have received LMCC after 1/1/78
Wyoming	Yes	Yes	

Abbreviations

ACGME—Accreditation Council for Graduate Medical Education

GME—graduate medical education

LMCC—certification by the Licentiate of the Medical Council of Canada

Note: *All information should be verified with the licensing board; licenses based on endorsement are granted to those physicians meeting all state requirements.*

Initial Licensure of International Medical Graduates (IMGs)

All international medical graduates (IMGs) must hold a certificate from the Educational Commission for Foreign Medical Graduates (ECFMG) examination before taking Step 3 of the United States Medical Licensing Examination (USMLE). (For more information on the ECFMG certificate, see page 104.)

Twenty-two boards maintain and/or use a list of approved/unapproved foreign medical schools for initial licensure decisions; several states use the list of schools from the California board (Table 9). In addition, about half of the boards require IMG candidates for endorsement of licensure to have graduated from a state-approved foreign medical school (see Table 5, column 3).

Thirty-nine states will endorse for licensure the Licentiate of the Medical Council of Canada (LMCC) when held by an IMG.

Twenty-three state boards allow IMGs to take USMLE Step 3 before they have had GME in a US or Canadian hospital (although some of these states require that a candidate be enrolled in a GME program). All states, however, require at least 1 year of GME for licensure, and 28 states require 3 years. Candidates are not awarded a license until they undertake the required GME in the United States and meet other board requirements (e.g., an ECFMG certificate, personal interview, payment of fees).

Fifth Pathway

In 1971, the AMA established the Fifth Pathway, a program for US citizens studying abroad at foreign medical schools. The program requires that participants have

1. Completed, in an accredited US college or university, undergraduate premedical work of a quality acceptable for matriculation in an accredited US medical school, evaluated by measures such as college grade point average and scores on the Medical College Admission Test

2. Studied medicine in a foreign medical school located outside the United States, including Puerto Rico, and Canada that is listed in the *International Medical Education Directory*, available on the ECFMG Web site at *www.ecfmg.org* and developed and maintained by the Foundation for Advancement of International Medical Education and Research (FAIMER[SM]), a nonprofit foundation of the ECFMG

3. Completed all formal requirements for a diploma of the foreign medical school except internship and/or social service (Those who have completed all the formal graduation requirements of the foreign medical school, including internship and/or social service, and are consequently eligible to apply for ECFMG certification, are not eligible for the Fifth Pathway program.)

If the aforementioned criteria are met, the candidate may substitute the Fifth Pathway program for internship and/or social service in the foreign country. After receiving a Fifth Pathway certificate from an accredited US medical school, these US citizens are eligible to enter the first year of GME in the United States.

In 52 jurisdictions (exceptions are Guam and the Virgin Islands), individuals who hold Fifth Pathway certificates (but not the ECFMG certificate) are eligible for licensure. Fifth Pathway certificate holders must pass Steps 1 and 2 of the USMLE before entering a GME program accredited by the Accreditation Council for Graduate Medical Education (ACGME).

Note: As of June 30, 2009, through action of the AMA Council on Medical Education, the Fifth Pathway has been discontinued. The Council no longer supports the Fifth Pathway as a mechanism for eligibility to enter the first year of ACGME-accredited graduate medical education programs. The AMA will continue to maintain record of former graduates of Fifth Pathway programs, but will no longer add records of individuals completing a year of supervised clinical education at an LCME-accredited medical school in the United States after July 1, 2009, although entrants beginning in January 2009 will be included.

Additional Notes for Specific Licensing Jurisdictions

California—The state maintains lists of both recognized and disapproved schools, available at:
   www.mbc.ca.gov/applicant/schools_recognized.html
   www.mbc.ca.gov/applicant/schools_unapproved.html

Neither education completed at nor diplomas issued by the 10 schools currently on the disapproved list will be accepted toward meeting the requirements for training and/or licensure in the state. The following list shows the name of medical school and date disapproved.

1. CETEC University, Santo Domingo (closed)
   May 19, 1983

2. CIFAS University, Santo Domingo (closed)
November 16, 1984

3. UTESA University, Santo Domingo
July 13, 1985 (disapproval reaffirmed 02-07-97)

4. World University, Santo Domingo (closed)
December 1, 1989

5. Spartan Health Sciences University, St. Lucia
June 13, 1985

6. University of Health Sciences Antigua, St. John's
July 28, 1995

7. Universidad Eugenio Maria de Hostos (UNIREMHOS),
Dominican Republic
November 1, 1996

8. Universidad Federico Henriquez y Carvajal, Dom. Rep.
July 31, 1998

9. St. Matthew's University, Grand Cayman
February 18, 2005

10. Kigezi International School of Medicine, Cambridge,
England and Uganda
November 2, 2007

Florida—ECFMG certificate required for licensure if a candidate is not a graduate of a foreign medical school approved by the Florida Board of Medicine (none has yet been approved).

Idaho—No list of approved foreign medical schools is maintained, but for IMGs applying for licensure, such schools must have been in existence for at least 15 years from the date of application for Idaho licensure.

Kansas—Licensure applicants must have graduated from a school approved by the Board. If the school has not been approved by the Board, an applicant may still be eligible for a license if the school has not been disapproved and has been in operation (date instruction started) for not less than 15 years.

Schools approved by the Board are:

1. All schools accredited by the Liaison Committee for Medical Eduction (LCME)

2. Universidad Autonoma de Guadalajara, Mexico

3. Aga Khan, Pakistan

4. American University of the Caribbean, Montserat

5. SABA University, Netherlands (for graduates who matriculated at the school from and after January 1, 2002)

6. Ziauddin Medical School (temporarily approved from 7-1-08 through 6-30-11 for postgraduate permits only)

7. Kamineni Institute of Medical Sciences (temporarily approved from 7-1-08 through 6-30-12 for postgraduate permits only)

Schools unapproved (neither approved or disapproved) by the Board are:

1. SABA University, Netherlands (for graduates who matriculated at the school before 2002)

Applicants from any school disapproved by the Board are not eligible for licensure. The schools are:

1. UTESA University, Santo Domingo

2. Universidad Eugenio Maria de Hostos (UNIREMHOS), Dominican Republic

3. St. Matthew's University, Grand Cayman

For more information, see:
www.ksbha.org/medicalschoolsapprovedunapproved.html

Maine—GME taken in Canada or the British Isles (accredited by a national body deemed equivalent to ACGME) may be considered qualifying on an individual basis.

Maryland—In addition to 2 years of ACGME- or RCPSC-accredited GME required for licensure, 1 year of GME required if a candidate failed any part of an examination three times; no more than three failures permitted.

Mississippi—ABMS board certification required for candidates who completed the Fifth Pathway.

Nevada—A formal list of approved/unapproved medical schools is not maintained, but the board does have an internal list of questionable medical schools.

New Jersey—An individual's educational experience must meet certain eligibility requirements.

North Carolina—Less than 3 years of GME may be accepted if applicant has completed at least 1 year of approved GME and is certified by an ABMS or AOA specialty board.

North Dakota—Three years of US or Canadian GME is required for licensure; if a candidate has not completed

3 years of GME but has met all other licensing requirements and has completed 1 year of GME in the United States or Canada in a board-approved program, and if the board finds that the candidate has other professional experience and training substantially equivalent to the second and third years of GME, the candidate may be deemed eligible for licensure (upon passing SPEX or ABMS board certification).

Oregon—IMG candidates for licensure must have completed at least 3 years of progressive GME in not more than two specialties in not more than two US or Canadian hospitals accredited for such training.

Pennsylvania—The board will grant unrestricted license by endorsement to a candidate who does not meet standard requirements if the candidate has achieved cumulative qualifications that are endorsed by the board as being equivalent to the standard license requirements.

South Carolina—ABMS/AOA board certification required for candidates who completed the Fifth Pathway.

South Dakota—No list of approved/unapproved foreign medical schools is maintained; decisions made on a case-by-case basis.

Texas—Canadian graduates of LCME-accredited schools are considered equivalent to US graduates for educational and post-graduate training requirements.

Table 9
Initial Licensure of International Medical Graduates (IMGs)

	Accepts Fifth Pathway	Maintains/ Uses List of Approved Foreign Med Schools	Endorses Canadian Certificate (LMCC) Held by an IMG	Amount of Accredited US or Canadian GME Required	
				...to Take USMLE Step 3	...for Licensure
Alabama	Yes	Yes	Yes	2 yrs (must be in 3rd yr of GME)	3 yrs
Alaska	Yes	Yes	Yes	1 yr	3 yrs
Arizona	Yes	No	Yes	6 mos	3 yrs
Arkansas	Yes	Yes (CA list)	Yes	None	3 yrs (1 if currently enrolled in prgm at U of Arkansas for Med Sci)
California*	Yes	Yes	Yes	None	2 yrs (including 4 mos general med)
Colorado	Yes	Yes	No	3 yrs	3 yrs
Connecticut	Yes	Yes (WHO)	Yes	None	2 yrs
Delaware	Yes	No	No	1 yr	3 yrs
DC	Yes	No	Yes	3 yrs	3 yrs
Florida*	Yes	No	No	None	2 yrs
Georgia	Yes	Yes (CA list)	Yes	1-3 yrs	3 yrs (1 yr prior to July 1, 1985)
Guam	No	No	No	2 yrs	3 yrs
Hawaii	Yes	No	No	1 yr (must be in 2nd yr of pgm)	2 yrs
Idaho*	Yes	No	No	2 yrs, 9 mos	3 yrs
Illinois	Yes	No	Yes	1 yr	1 yr (entered GME pre-1988); 2 yrs (entered GME post-1988)
Indiana	Yes	Yes	Yes	2 yrs	2 yrs
Iowa	Yes	Yes	Yes (with valid Canadian provincial license and fulfillment of all other licensure requirements)	7 mos (or enrollment in GME pgm approved by board at time of application for Step 3)	2 yrs AOA-, ACGME-, RCPSC-, or CFPC-accredited GME
Kansas*	Yes	Yes	Yes	2 yrs (or enrollment in GME program in Kansas)	2 yrs
Kentucky	Yes	No	Yes	1 yr	2 yrs
Louisiana	Yes	Yes (WHO)	No	None	3 yrs (Fifth Pathway may be counted as 1 yr of required GME)
Maine*	Yes	Yes (IMED)	Yes	1 yr	3 yrs
Maryland*	Yes	No	Yes	None (1 yr if 3 fails on any Step)	2 yrs ACGME- or RCPSC-accredited GME (as of Oct. 1, 2000)
Massachusetts	Yes	No	Yes	1 yr	2 yrs
Michigan	Yes	No	Yes (with valid Canadian license)	6 mos	2 yrs
Minnesota	Yes	Yes (WHO)	Yes	None (must be in GME program)	2 yrs
Mississippi*	Yes	No	No	1 yr	3 yrs (or 1 yr plus ABMS certification)
Missouri	Yes	No	No	3 yrs	3 yrs
Montana	Yes	Yes	No	1 yr (plus ECFMG)	3 yrs (or ABMS/AOA certification)
Nebraska	Yes	No	Yes	None	3 yrs
Nevada*	Yes	No	Yes	None	3 yrs
New Hampshire	Yes	No	Yes	1 yr	2 yrs
New Jersey*	Yes	Yes (WHO)*	No	1 yr	3 yrs (1 yr if medical school completed before July 1, 1985); 2 yrs, and contract for yr 3, if graduated after July 1, 2003

(continued on next page)

Table 9 (continued)
Initial Licensure of International Medical Graduates (IMGs)

	Accepts Fifth Pathway	Maintains/ Uses List of Approved Foreign Med Schools	Endorses Canadian Certificate (LMCC) Held by an IMG	Amount of Accredited US or Canadian GME Required	
				...to Take USMLE Step 3	...for Licensure
New Mexico	Yes	Yes (CA list)	No	1 yr	2 yrs
New York	Yes	No	Yes (with valid Canadian provincial license and fulfillment of all other licensure requirements)	None	3 yrs
North Carolina*	Yes	No	Yes	None	3 yrs
North Dakota*	Yes	Yes (CA list)	Yes	1 yr (none if enrolled in-state)	3 yrs
Ohio	Yes	No	Yes	9 mos	2 yrs (through the 2nd-yr level)
Oklahoma	Yes	No	Yes	None	2 yrs
Oregon*	Yes	Yes (CA list)	Yes	None (must be in GME program)	3 yrs
Pennsylvania*	Yes	No	Yes (if passed after 5/70 and in English)	None	3 yrs (1 yr if GME taken in US before July 1987)
Puerto Rico	Yes		Yes	None	1 yr
Rhode Island	Yes	Yes (WHO)	Yes (with valid Canadian provincial license and fulfillment of all other licensure requirements)	1 yr	3 yrs
South Carolina*	Yes	No	Yes	3 yrs	3 yrs
South Dakota*	Yes	No	Yes	1 yr	Completion of residency (1 yr if US GME taken before 7/87)
Tennessee	Yes	Yes	Yes	1 yr	3 yrs
Texas*	Yes	Yes	No (but accepts LMCC examination as licensing examination)	None	3 yrs
Utah	Yes	No	No	None	2 yrs
Vermont	Yes	Yes (CA list)	Yes	7 mos	3 yrs
Virgin Islands	No	No	No	Not applicable	1 yr US GME
Virginia	Yes	No	Yes	None	2 yrs
Washington	Yes	No	Yes (if passed after 12/69)	1 yr (or enrollment in GME program)	2 yrs (1 yr if medical school completed before July 28, 1985)
West Virginia	Yes	No	Yes	None	3 yrs (or 1 yr plus ABMS cert.)
Wisconsin	Yes	No	Yes (if passed after 12/77)	1 yr	1 yr
Wyoming	Yes	No	Yes	1 yr	1 yr

Abbreviations

ABMS—American Board of Medical Specialties (ABMS)
ACGME—Accreditation Council for Graduate Medical Education
AOA—American Osteopathic Association
CFPC—College of Family Physicians of Canada
ECFMG—Educational Commission for Foreign Medical Graduates
GME—graduate medical education
IMED—International Medical Education Directory
IMG—international medical graduate
LMCC—Licentiate of the Medical Council of Canada
RCPSC—Royal College of Physicians and Surgeons of Canada
USMLE—United States Medical Licensing Examination
WHO—World Health Organization

* Refer to introductory text to this table for more information on this state's regulations.

Note: *All information should be verified with the licensing board; licenses are granted to those physicians meeting all state requirements—at the discretion of the board.*

Medical Student Clerkship Regulations

For purposes of this publication, a clerkship is defined as clinical education provided to medical students. Twenty states evaluate the quality of clinical clerkships in connection with an application for licensure. In most states, clerkships for US medical students must take place in hospitals affiliated with medical schools accredited by the Liaison Committee on Medical Education (LCME). Eleven of these 20 states have additional and/or more specific bases for evaluation, which are particularly relevant for students of non-LCME-accredited medical schools in the Caribbean, the majority of which complete their clinical clerkships in US hospitals and teaching institutions.

For example, Texas (as noted below) requires that the clerkship(s) must be performed in a hosital or teaching institution sponsoring or participating in a graduate medical education (GME) program accredited, at the time the applicant performed the clerkship, by the ACGME, AOA, or the board in the *same subject* (e.g., the *exact same specialty or subspecialty*). Required core (or fundamental) clinical clerkships are:

- Internal medicine
- Obstetrics-gynecology
- Pediatrics
- Psychiatry
- Family medicine
- Surgery

Thirteen boards regulate clerkships provided in their states to students of foreign medical schools (including US citizens studying medicine in foreign schools). Of these, Maryland, Pennsylvania, and Puerto Rico forbid such clerkships. For purposes of licensure, 21 states accept only those clerkships completed in hospital departments with ACGME-accredited programs. Nine states have additional regulations.

Additional Notes for Specific Licensing Jurisdictions

California—Students of foreign medical schools may complete up to 18 of 72 required weeks in nonapproved clerkships outside of California.

Florida—Rules on clinical clerkships for international medical graduates adopted by the Florida Board before October 1986 do not apply to any graduate who had already completed a clinical clerkship or who had begun a clinical clerkship, as long as the clerkship was completed within 3 years.

A foreign medical school must be registered with the Florida Department of Education for its students to perform clinical clerkships in Florida.

Michigan—Specific clerkships are required (only for MDs).

New Jersey—For students from foreign medical schools (i.e., non-LCME or AOA-accredited) who complete clinical clerkships in the US, the core clerkships (internal medicine, obstetrics-gynecology, pediatrics, psychiatry, and surgery) must be completed (minimum of 4 weeks in each) at facilities that maintain an ACGME- or AOA-accredited residency program in the specific specialty.

Pennsylvania—Students of foreign medical schools are not permitted to engage in clinical clerkships within Pennsylvania.

Texas—Clerkships must be performed 1) as a student in an accredited medical or osteopathic school, or 2) in a hospital or teaching institution sponsoring or participating in a GME program accredited by the ACGME, the AOA, or the board in the same specialty or subspecialty as the medical or osteopathic medical education. The only exception is for applicants who are ABMS or AOA Bureau of Osteopathic Specialists specialty board certified.

Table 10
Medical Student Clerkship Regulations

	Evaluates the Quality of Clinical Clerkships in Connection with a Licensure Application	Regulation of Clerkships Provided to Students of Foreign Medical Schools			
		Regulates Clerkships Provided by Hospitals	Forbids Clerkships for Students of Foreign Med. Schools	Accepts Clerkships Only in Hospital Departments with ACGME-accredited Programs	Has Additional Regulations
Alabama	Yes			Yes	
Alaska					
Arizona					
Arkansas	Yes†	Yes		Yes	
California*	Yes†	Yes		Yes	Yes
Colorado					
Connecticut	Yes†	Yes		Yes	
Delaware	Yes	Yes		Yes	
DC					
Florida*	Yes	Yes		Yes	Yes
Georgia	Yes†			Yes	
Guam	Yes			Yes	
Hawaii					
Idaho					
Illinois					
Indiana				Yes	
Iowa					
Kansas					
Kentucky	Yes			Yes	
Louisiana					
Maine				Yes	
Maryland		Yes	Yes		Yes
Massachusetts	Yes†	Yes		Yes	Yes
Michigan*					Yes
Minnesota					
Mississippi					
Missouri					
Montana					
Nebraska					
Nevada				Yes	
New Hampshire					
New Jersey*	Yes†	Yes		Yes	Yes
New Mexico	Yes†				
New York	Yes†	Yes		Yes	Yes
North Carolina					
North Dakota					
Ohio					
Oklahoma				Yes	
Oregon	Yes	Yes		Yes	
Pennsylvania*	Yes†	Yes	Yes	Yes	

(continued on next page)

Table 10 (continued)
Medical Student Clerkship Regulations

	Evaluates the Quality of Clinical Clerkships in Connection with a Licensure Application	Regulation of Clerkships Provided to Students of Foreign Medical Schools			Has Additional Regulations
		Regulates Clerkships Provided by Hospitals	Forbids Clerkships for Students of Foreign Med. Schools	Accepts Clerkships Only in Hospital Departments with ACGME-accredited Programs	
Puerto Rico	Yes	Yes	Yes		
Rhode Island	Yes			Yes	
South Carolina					
South Dakota					
Tennessee					
Texas*	Yes†	Yes		Yes	Yes
Utah					
Vermont					
Virgin Islands					
Virginia	Yes†			Yes	
Washington					
West Virginia					
Wisconsin	No	No	No	No	No
Wyoming	Yes				Yes
Total	**20**	**13**	**2**	**21**	**9**

* Refer to introductory text to this table for more information on this state's regulations.

† In many cases, clerkships must take place in hospitals affiliated with LCME-accredited medical schools or ACGME-accredited residency programs. These states require additional and/or more specific criteria for evaluation.

Abbreviation

ACGME—Accreditation Council for Graduate Medical Education

Note: *All information should be verified with the licensing board; medical licenses are granted to those physicians meeting all state requirements—at the discretion of the board.*

Additional Policies Concerning International Medical Graduates (IMGs) and Doctors of Osteopathic Medicine (DOs)

A number of state medical boards have additional graduate medical education (GME) and specialty certificate policies for international medical graduates (IMGs). Fourteen states have requirements for appointment to GME programs other than requiring an Educational Commission for Foreign Medical Graduates (ECFMG) certificate or a limited license.

Seven boards—Connecticut, Maine, Nebraska, Ohio, Oklahoma, Rhode Island, and Texas—indicated that GME completed in foreign countries other than Canada may be considered for credit toward a license. Specialty certificates of foreign boards, such as the Royal College of Physicians in the United Kingdom, may be accepted for credit toward a license in 11 states.

Thirty-nine medical boards accept GME accredited by the Accreditation Council for Graduate Medical Education (ACGME) for licensure of osteopathic medical graduates.

Additional Notes for Specific Licensing Jurisdictions

Maine—The board may accept GME completed in England, Scotland, and Ireland for credit toward a license, if it is accepted by the specialty board as meeting board eligibility in the United States and notified via certified letter.

Pennsylvania—IMGs seeking appointment to a GME program need a passing score on United States Medical Licensing Examination (USMLE) Steps 1 and 2 (or National Board of Medical Examiners [NBME] Parts I and II or Federation Licensing Examination [FLEX] Component 1) for graduate year 2 medical education; for graduate year 3 and beyond, all parts of USMLE (or NBME or FLEX) are required.

Wisconsin—Temporary educational permit is required of IMGs for a second year of GME (and beyond), unless IMG has a permanent license. Board may accept training in lieu of graduate medical education by waiver.

Table 11
Additional Policies Concerning International Medical Graduates (IMGs) and Doctors of Osteopathic Medicine (DOs)

	Has State Board Requirements for Appointment to GME Program Other Than ECFMG Certificate or Limited License	May Accept GME Completed in Foreign Countries Other Than Canada for Credit Toward a License	May Accept Specialty Certificates of Foreign Boards (e.g., Royal College of Physicians of the United Kingdom) for Credit Toward a License	Osteopathic Medical Graduates	
				ACGME-Accredited GME Accepted	State Osteopathic Board Handles Licensure
Alabama				Yes	
Alaska	Yes (residency permit required)				
Arizona	Yes (residency permit required)				Yes
Arkansas				Yes	
California	Yes	No	No		Yes
Colorado				Yes	
Connecticut	Yes (residency intern permit required)	Yes	Yes	Yes	
Delaware					
DC				Yes	
Florida					Yes
Georgia				Yes	
Guam					
Hawaii				Yes	
Idaho				Yes	
Illinois				Yes	
Indiana				Yes	
Iowa				Yes	
Kansas	Yes (residency permit required, and unapproved school must have been in existence at least 15 yrs)			Yes	
Kentucky	Yes (residency permit required for 2nd yr)			Yes	
Louisiana	Yes (passage of FLEX/NBME/USMLE)			Yes	
Maine*		Yes	Yes	Yes	Yes
Maryland				Yes	
Massachusetts				Yes	
Michigan	Yes (certification of medical education)				Yes
Minnesota	Yes (residency intern permit required)			Yes	
Mississippi				Yes	
Missouri	Yes			Yes	
Montana				Yes	
Nebraska		Yes		Yes	
Nevada	Yes				Yes
New Hampshire				Yes	
New Jersey	Yes (residency intern permit required)			Yes	
New Mexico					Yes
New York			Yes	Yes	
North Carolina				Yes	
North Dakota			Yes	Yes	
Ohio		Yes	Yes	Yes	

(continued on next page)

Table 11 (continued)
Additional Policies Concerning International Medical Graduates (IMGs) and Doctors of Osteopathic Medicine (DOs)

	Has State Board Requirements for Appointment to GME Program Other Than ECFMG Certificate or Limited License	May Accept GME Completed in Foreign Countries Other Than Canada for Credit Toward a License	May Accept Specialty Certificates of Foreign Boards (e.g., Royal College of Physicians of the United Kingdom) for Credit Toward a License	Osteopathic Medical Graduates	
				ACGME-Accredited GME Accepted	State Osteopathic Board Handles Licensure
Oklahoma		Yes	Yes		Yes
Oregon				Yes	
Pennsylvania*	Yes		Yes		Yes
Puerto Rico					
Rhode Island		Yes (UK only)	Yes; may accept certificates of boards in England, Scotland, and Ireland	Yes	
South Carolina				Yes	
South Dakota				Yes	
Tennessee			Yes; specialty board must be AMA-recognized		Yes
Texas		Yes		Yes	
Utah				Yes	Yes
Vermont	Yes		Yes; specialty board must be recognized by ABMS, RCPSC, or CFPC		Yes
Virgin Islands					
Virginia				Yes	
Washington				Yes	Yes
West Virginia				Yes	Yes
Wisconsin*			No	Yes	
Wyoming			Yes (at board's discretion)	Yes	
Total	**14**	**7**	**11**	**39**	**13**

Abbreviations

ABMS—American Board of Medical Specialties (ABMS)
ACGME—Accreditation Council for Graduate Medical Education
ECFMG—Educational Commission for Foreign Medical Graduates
CFPC—College of Family Physicians of Canada
FLEX—Federation Licensing Examination
GME—graduate medical education
NBME—certificate of the National Board of Medical Examiners
RCPSC—Royal College of Physicians and Surgeons of Canada
USMLE—United States Medical Licensing Examination

* Refer to introductory text to this table for more information on this state's regulations.

Note: *All information should be verified with the licensing board; medical licenses are granted to those physicians meeting all state requirements—at the discretion of the board.*

Accredited Subspecialties and Nonaccredited Fellowships That Satisfy Graduate Medical Education Requirements for Licensure

Both the AMA and the Accreditation Council for Graduate Medical Education (ACGME) define a residency as graduate medical education (GME) that takes place in any of the medical specialties with ACGME Program Requirements (e.g., internal medicine, pediatrics, surgery). Beginning in 2000, the ACGME has used the term *fellowship* to denote GME in ACGME-accredited subspecialty programs (e.g., cardiovascular disease, hand surgery, rheumatology) that is beyond the requirements for eligibility for first board certification in the discipline.

All state medical boards accept residency education in specialty programs accredited by the ACGME as satisfying their GME requirements for licensure. Fifty-one jurisdictions—all except Arkansas, Michigan (DO), and Puerto Rico—accept residency education in subspecialty programs accredited by ACGME as satisfying their GME requirements for licensure (Table 12).

Ten boards accept clinical fellowships not accredited by ACGME, and three boards—Hawaii, New York, and North Carolina—may accept research fellowships not accredited by ACGME to satisfy the GME requirement for licensure.

For more information on the ACGME, see page 129.

Table 12
Accredited Subspecialties and Nonaccredited Fellowships That Satisfy Graduate Medical Education Requirements for Licensure

	Accepts Subspecialty GME Accredited by ACGME	Accepts Clinical Fellowships *Not* Accredited by ACGME	Accepts Research Fellowships *Not* Accredited by ACGME
Alabama	Yes		
Alaska	Yes		
Arizona	Yes		
Arkansas	No		
California MD and DO	Yes		
Colorado	Yes		
Connecticut	Yes		
Delaware	Yes		
DC	Yes		
Florida	Yes		
Georgia	Yes	Yes	
Guam	Yes		
Hawaii	Yes	Yes (with board approval)	Yes (with board approval)
Idaho	Yes		
Illinois	Yes		
Indiana	Yes		
Iowa	Yes		
Kansas	Yes		
Kentucky	Yes		
Louisiana	Yes		
Maine	Yes		
Maryland	Yes	Yes (with board approval)	
Massachusetts	Yes		
Michigan	Yes		
Michigan DO	Only if AOA-accredited		
Minnesota	Yes		
Mississippi	Yes		
Missouri	Yes	Yes	
Montana	Yes		
Nebraska	Yes		
Nevada	Yes		
New Hampshire	Yes		
New Jersey	Yes		
New Mexico	Yes		
New York	Yes	Yes	Yes
North Carolina	Yes	Yes (with board approval)	Yes (with board approval)
North Dakota	Yes		
Ohio	Yes	Yes (with board approval)	
Oklahoma	Yes		
Oregon	Yes		
Pennsylvania	Yes		
Puerto Rico	No		
Rhode Island	Yes	Yes (with board approval)	
South Carolina	Yes		
South Dakota	Yes		

(continued on next page)

Table 12 (continued)

Accredited Subspecialties and Nonaccredited Fellowships That Satisfy Graduate Medical Education Requirements for Licensure

	Accepts Subspecialty GME Accredited by ACGME	Accepts Clinical Fellowships *Not* Accredited by ACGME	Accepts Research Fellowships *Not* Accredited by ACGME
Tennessee	Yes		
Texas	Yes	Yes (if board-approved)	
Utah	Yes	Yes (if combined with an ACGME-accredited program)	
Vermont	Yes		
Virgin Islands	Yes		
Virginia	Yes		
Washington MD and DO	Yes		
West Virginia	Yes		
Wisconsin	Yes		
Wyoming	Yes		
Total	**51**	**10**	**3**

Abbreviations

ACGME—Accreditation Council for Graduate Medical Education
AOA—American Osteopathic Association
GME—graduate medical education

* Refer to introductory text to this table for more information on this state's regulations.

Note: *All information should be verified with licensing board; medical licenses are granted to those physicians meeting all state requirements—at the discretion of the board.*

Licensure Requirement Exemptions for Eminent Physicians and Medical School Faculty

Eighteen boards license physicians through recognition of eminence in medical education or medical practice (Table 13). For example, Maryland, one of the jurisdictions that licenses physicians through this mechanism, defines "Conceded eminence and authority in the profession" as "significant teaching, research, and achievement in a field of medicine recognized by the Board" (see *www.mbp.state.md.us/forms/concede.pdf*)

In Maryland, applicants seeking licensure by eminence must meet at least three of the following qualifications:

1. *Within 10 years before the application, have published original results of clinical research in a medical journal listed in the Index Medicus or in an equivalent scholarly publication, and have submitted these articles to the Board in English or in a foreign language with verifiable, certified translations in English;*

2. *Have held an appointment at a medical school approved by the LCME or at any medical school listed in the World Health Organization directory at the level of associate or full professor, or its equivalent, for at least 5 years;*

3. *Within 10 years before the application, have developed a treatment modality, surgical technique, or other verified original contribution to the field of medicine, which is attested to by the dean of a school of medicine in the State or by the director of the National Institutes of Health;*

4. *Have actively practiced medicine cumulatively for 15 years, which may include up to 5 years sabbatical during which the applicant was involved in research; and*

5. *Be a member in good standing of a board of the American Board of Medical Specialties or other equivalent specialty board.*

Physicians appointed to a medical school faculty are excused from the graduate medical education (GME) requirement for limited licensure in 21 states and from the examination requirement for limited licensure or teaching certification in 20 states. These faculty appointees would, however, receive a limited license or similar credential.

Table 13
Licensure Requirement Exemptions for Eminent Physicians and Medical School Faculty

	License Physicians Through Recognition of Eminence in Medical Education or Practice	Physicians Appointed to a Medical Faculty Are Excused From...		Notes/Comments
		...the GME Requirement for Limited Licensure	...the Examination Requirement for Limited Licensure	
Alabama		Yes	Yes	
Alaska				
Arizona				
Arkansas				
California DO	Yes	Yes	Yes	
California MD	Yes	Yes	Yes	1-yr medical faculty certificate, for practice only at the medical school or a formally affiliated teaching hospital.
Colorado	Yes	Yes	Yes	Distinguished foreign physicians are invited to serve on faculty.
Connecticut		Yes	Yes	
Delaware				
DC	Yes			
Florida		Yes	Yes	Physicians appointed to a medical faculty are eligible for a special license, with which they may practice only at the designated facility/institution.
Georgia		Yes	Yes	Physicians appointed to a medical faculty are excused from the GME requirement for limited licensure for teaching only.
Guam				
Hawaii				
Idaho				
Illinois				
Indiana				
Iowa	Yes	Yes	Yes	Physicians appointed to a medical faculty are eligible for a special license, with which they may practice only at the designated facility/institution. Time spent on a special license can be applied to the GME requirements for permanent licensure.
Kansas				
Kentucky	Yes	Yes	Yes	Physicians appointed to a medical faculty are eligible for a special license, with which they may practice only at the designated facility/institution.
Louisiana	Yes	Yes	Yes	A physician licensed through recognition of eminence in medical education must be approved as a tenured professor or associate/assistant professor by a Louisiana medical school.
Maine				
Maryland	Yes	Yes	Yes	
Massachusetts				
Michigan (MD and DO)	Yes (limited)	Yes	Yes	Only IMGs with an appointment to an approved program.
Minnesota				
Mississippi				
Missouri	Yes		Yes	
Montana	Yes			An IMG seeking a restricted license must have published in an English-language, peer-reviewed medical journal.
Nebraska				
Nevada	Yes			
New Hampshire	Yes			A courtesy license for educational purposes is provided to eminent physicians under limited circumstances.

(continued on next page)

Table 13 (continued)
Licensure Requirement Exemptions for Eminent Physicians and Medical School Faculty

	License Physicians Through Recognition of Eminence in Medical Education or Practice	Physicians Appointed to a Medical Faculty Are Excused From...		Notes/Comments
		...the GME Requirement for Limited Licensure	...the Examination Requirement for Limited Licensure	
New Jersey				
New Mexico				
New York				
North Carolina	Yes	Yes	Yes	Also excused from ECFMG certification requirement.
North Dakota				
Ohio		Yes	Yes	Physicians appointed to a medical faculty are eligible for visiting medical faculty certificate, with which they may practice only at the school or teaching hospitals affiliated with the school. This nonrenewable certificate is valid 3 yrs or duration of the appointment, whichever is shorter.
Oklahoma				
Oregon		Yes		IMGs not eligible for licensure may be granted a Limited License, Medical Faculty (LL,MF) if appointed to a full-time medical school faculty position under direction of the department head. LL,MF may be granted and renewed for a total of 4 yrs, during which applicant must pass the USMLE or have passed FLEX or the National Boards. The physician would then be eligible for licensure.
Pennsylvania DO				
Pennsylvania MD	Yes	Yes	.	Physicians appointed to a medical faculty are eligible for a visiting medical faculty certificate, with which they may practice only at the school or teaching hospitals affiliated with the school. This nonrenewable certificate is valid 1 yr or duration of the appointment, whichever is shorter.
Puerto Rico				
Rhode Island	Yes	Yes	Yes	Distinguished foreign physicians recommended by the medical school dean may serve on faculty; academic limited registration may be renewed for a maximum of 5 yrs.
South Carolina				
South Dakota				
Tennessee		Yes	Yes	
Texas	Yes	See note	See note	There are several types of limited licenses, each with different requirements and characteristics.
Utah				
Vermont		Yes	Yes	
Virgin Islands				
Virginia	Yes	Yes	Yes	
Washington				
West Virginia		Yes	Yes	
Wisconsin				
Wyoming				Exemption granted at Board's discretion.
Total	**18**	**21**	**20**	

Abbreviations

ECFMG—Educational Commission for Foreign Medical Graduates

FLEX—Federation Licensing Examination

GME—graduate medical education

IMG—international medical graduate

USMLE—United States Medical Licensing Examination

Note: *All information should be verified with licensing board; medical licenses are granted to those physicians meeting all state requirements—at the discretion of the board.*

Teaching (Visiting Professor) Licenses

Forty jurisdictions issue teaching (visiting professor) licenses, with fees ranging from $0 to $400 (Table 14).

These permits are granted for various periods of time; for example, Arizona (both the MD and DO boards) offer a teaching license valid for 1 year, which may be renewed for up to 4 years; California awards renewable certificates of registration for 1 to 3 years; Illinois offers visiting professor permits valid for up to 2 years; Oregon offers a 1-year limited license for either visiting professors or medical faculty that can be renewed for 1 additional year or 3 additional years, respectively.

Awarding of these licenses may be contingent on certain requirements, depending on the given jurisdiction. For example, Washington state requires 1) a letter of nomination by the dean of the University of Washington medical school or CEO of a hospital or other appropriate health care facility and 2) proof of current licensure in another state or country.

Table 14
Teaching (Visiting Professor) Licenses

	Teaching (Visiting Professor) License Granted	Notes
Alabama	Yes	
Alaska		
Arizona	Yes, $100	Education teaching permit, granted for 5 days, $100. Teaching licenses, within Board-approved medical school or GME program, $225; valid 1 yr and may be renewed for up to 4 yrs.
Arizona DO	Yes, $318	Education teaching permit, granted for 5 days, $106.
Arkansas	Yes, $400	Education license must be renewed annually.
California	Yes	Renewable certificates of registration are awarded on an individual basis for 1 to 3 yrs to physicians who do not immediately meet licensure requirements and who have been offered full-time teaching positions in California medical schools. Biennially renewable faculty permits are awarded on an individual basis to academically eminent physicians for whom the medical school has assumed direct responsibility. The holder may practice medicine only within the sponsoring medical school and affiliated institutions.
California DO		
Colorado	Yes, $100	
Connecticut	Yes, $0	
Delaware		
DC		
Florida	Yes, $100	A visiting faculty certificate, valid for 180 days, is granted to MDs/DOs who are graduates of an accredited medical school or its equivalent and hold a valid current license to practice medicine in another US jurisdiction. The certificate authorizes practice only in conjunction with teaching duties at an accredited Florida medical/osteopathic school or in its main teaching hospitals. No more than three physicians per year per institution may hold this certificate; the certificate can be granted to a physician only once in a given 5-yr period.
Florida DO	Yes, $400	(See above note)
Georgia	Yes	Teacher's license for faculty of approved Georgia medical schools.
Guam		
Hawaii		
Hawaii DO		
Idaho		
Illinois	Yes	Visiting professor permits for a maximum of 2 yrs are issued to persons receiving faculty appointments to teach in either a medical or osteopathic school. Visiting physician permits for up to 180 days are issued to persons receiving an invitation or appointment to study, demonstrate, or perform a specific medical or osteopathic subject or technique in medical/osteopathic schools; hospitals; or facilities operated pursuant to the Ambulatory Surgical Treatment Center Act.
Indiana	Yes, $100	Visiting professor license granted to an institution for a specific physician to whom it has granted a visiting faculty appointment. Institution must certify the physician's qualifications; physician's practice limited to the institution for designated period not to exceed 1 yr.
Iowa	Yes	Special license or temporary license, depending on applicant's qualifications and the teaching activity in Iowa.
Kansas	Yes, $25	
Kentucky	Yes, $300	
Louisiana	Yes	License valid for specific period of time.
Maine	Yes, $0	
Maine DO	Yes, $50	
Maryland	Yes, $326	Limited 1-yr license for graduate teaching.
Massachusetts	Yes, $250	Temporary registration is issued to physicians who hold a temporary faculty appointment at a Massachusetts medical school, are substituting temporarily for a fully licensed Massachusetts physician, or are enrolled in a CME course that requires Massachusetts licensure.

(continued on next page)

Table 14 (continued)
Teaching (Visiting Professor) Licenses

	Teaching (Visiting Professor) License Granted	Notes
Michigan	Yes, $170	For teaching/research appointment at approved educational program.
Michigan DO	Yes, $170	For teaching/research appointment at approved educational program.
Minnesota		
Mississippi		
Missouri	Yes	
Montana		
Nebraska	Yes, $25	Temporary visiting faculty permits for medical school faculty.
Nevada		
Nevada DO	Yes, $200	Six-month maximum (considered special license).
New Hampshire	Yes, $75	
New Jersey		
New Mexico	Yes, $100	
New Mexico DO		
New York		
North Carolina	Yes, $150	Limited faculty license for faculty at medical schools and affiliated institutions.
North Dakota		
Ohio	Yes, $375	
Oklahoma		
Oklahoma DO		
Oregon	Yes, $185	Limited license (LL) is issued for Visiting Professor (VP) and Medical Faculty (MF). LL-VP is valid for a 1-yr teaching position and may be renewed for 1 additional yr. LL-MF is valid for a full-time faculty position offered by the dean of the medical school and may be renewed for 3 additional yrs.
Pennsylvania	Yes	Institutional license allows a qualified person to teach and/or practice medicine for a period of time not to exceed 3 yrs in one of the Commonwealth's medical colleges, its affiliates, or community hospitals. Temporary license allows the licensee to teach medicine and surgery or participate in a medical procedure necessary for the well-being of a specified patient within the Commonwealth. Applicants for a temporary license must hold an unrestricted license in another state, territory, possession, or country.
Pennsylvania DO		
Puerto Rico	Yes	
Rhode Island	Yes, $150	
South Carolina		
South Dakota		Teaching or visiting professor licenses, permits, or certificates are not issued.
Tennessee	Yes, $50	
Tennessee DO		
Texas	Yes, $110	
Utah		
Vermont		
Vermont DO		
Virgin Islands	Yes	
Virginia	Yes, $55	Limited license for fellowship and teaching positions.

(continued on next page)

Table 14 (continued)
Teaching (Visiting Professor) Licenses

	Teaching (Visiting Professor) License Granted	Notes
Washington	Yes (limited)	Teaching/research limited licenses may be granted for teaching (visiting professor) with 1) a letter of nomination by the dean of the University of Washington medical school or CEO of a hospital or other appropriate health care facility, and 2) proof of current licensure in another state or country.
Washington DO		
West Virginia	Yes, $150	Limited medical school faculty license.
West Virginia DO		
Wisconsin	Yes, $110	Visiting professor license for 2-yr period.
Wyoming		
Total	**40**	

Abbreviations

CME—continuing medical education

GME—graduate medical education

Note: *All information should be verified with licensing board; medical licenses are granted to those physicians meeting all state requirements—at the discretion of the board.*

Licensure and Reregistration Fees, Intervals, and Requirements

The National Board of Medical Examiners (NBME) administers United States Medical Licensing Examination (USMLE) Steps 1 and 2 to students and graduates of US and Canadian medical schools at test centers established by the NBME; application materials are usually available at these medical schools. The Educational Commission for Foreign Medical Graduates (ECFMG) administers USMLE Steps 1 and 2 to students and graduates of foreign medical schools; application materials are available only through the ECFMG.

Administration of USMLE Step 3 is the responsibility of the individual medical licensing jurisdictions. Step 3 application materials for physicians who have successfully completed Steps 1 and 2 are available from the medical licensing authorities or the Federation of State Medical Boards (FSMB), which administers the examination for all jurisdictions, except Florida, Guam, and the Virgin Islands. For more information on USMLE Step 3, call (800) USMLE XM—(800) 876-5396. Although the FSMB administers the examination, in five jurisdictions (Alabama, District of Columbia, Missouri, Puerto Rico, and Wisconsin) physicians apply for the examination directly via the state board rather than by way of the FSMB.

The fee for 2010 for USMLE Step 3 is $705; exceptions for are Iowa ($760), South Dakota ($860), and Vermont ($745).

For osteopathic physicians, the National Board of Osteopathic Medical Examiners (NBOME) administers the Comprehensive Osteopathic Medical Licensing Examination (COMLEX-USA) at various sites throughout the United States. For 2010, the Level 3 examination fee is $675.

In addition to these USMLE and COMLEX examination fees, most jurisdictions charge processing, application, and administrative fees; the average cost is $359. Including these fees, the average total cost of licensure by examination is $1,061 (Table 15).

Fees for licensure by endorsement, *including processing, application, and administrative fees*, average $392.

The majority of boards require physicians licensed in the state to reregister (or renew) their licenses every 1 or 2 years; five jurisdictions—Illinois, Michigan, Michigan DO, New Mexico, and Puerto Rico—have a 3-year reregistration interval. The average reregistration fee is $359, or $214 when calculated per year. Many states offer reduced fees for reregistration of inactive licenses (see Table 19 for more information).

Completion of a specified number of hours of continuing medical education (CME) is required for reregistration by 62 boards. See Table 16 for more information.

Additional Notes for Specific Licensing Jurisdictions

California—Endorsement fee includes a $442 processing fee, $51 fingerprinting fee, $25 mandatory loan repayment fee, and $808 licensing fee. Resident physician applicants are charged a reduced licensing fee of $416.

Illinois—Reregistration fee for nonresidents is $600. Penalty of $100 is charged if renewal is not submitted by July 31 in the year of renewal.

Maryland—Initial license $916 for IMGs. Reinstatement of lapsed license $626 or $726, depending on renewal year.

North Carolina—Criminal background check fee is $38.

Ohio—The Federation Credentials Verification Service (FCVS) is required of all physicians applying for Ohio licensure by either examination or endorsement. The applicable FCVS fee is in addition to the application fee paid to the medical board.

Texas—Initial applications are for licensure (not identified as examination or endorsement). The application fee is $885 and does not include any examination fees or criminal history check fees.

Washington—Note: These fees are nonrefundable.

- Impaired physician program fee on each application and for each year of the renewal period—$35
- University of Washington library fee per application or renewal—$25
- Late fee—$262
- Reissue expired license fee—$262

Wisconsin—Licensure re-registration application ($188) is required if license expired more than 5 years prior.

Table 15
Licensure, Endorsement, and Reregistration Fees, Intervals, and Requirements

	Examination							Licensure Reregistration			
	USMLE Step 3 Fee ($)	COMLEX Level 3 Fee ($)	Other Lic. Application Fees ($)	Total Cost ($)	Application to:		Endorsement Fees ($)	Registration Interval	Regular Fee ($)	CME Credits Required	Notes
					FSMB	NBOME					
Alabama	705		175	880	No		175	1 yr	200	Yes	
Alaska	705	.	840	1,545	Yes		250	2 yrs	590	Yes	$250: Application fee for licensure endorsement
Arizona	705		500	1,205	Yes		500	2 yrs	500	Yes	
Arizona DO		675	400	1,075		Yes	400	2 yrs	636	Yes	Biennial fee
Arkansas	705		400	1,105	Yes		400	1 yr	200	Yes	$100 processing fee
California*	705		442	1,147	Yes		1,326	2 yrs	808	Yes	Biennial fee; $51 fingerprint fee; $25 loan repayment fee
California DO		675	251	926		Yes	251	2 yrs	400	Yes	
Colorado	705		425	1,130	Yes		425	2 yrs	500		
Connecticut	705		450	1,155	Yes		450	1 yr	450	Yes	
Delaware	705		0	705	Yes			2 yrs	281	Yes	$61.50 criminal background check
DC	705		221	926	No		305	2 yrs	500	Yes	
Florida	705		815	1,520	Yes		500	2 yrs	429	Yes	$500 application fee for licensure
Florida DO		675	605	1,280		Yes	605	2 yrs	405	Yes	
Georgia	705		400	1,105	Yes		400	2 yrs	155	Yes	
Guam	705		400	1,105	Yes		400	2 yrs	250	Yes	
Hawaii	705	675	290	995	Yes	Yes	290	2 yrs	240	Yes	
Hawaii DO		675	400	1,075		Yes	400	2 yrs	190		
Idaho	705		0	705	Yes		400	1 or 2 yrs	200	Yes	Reregistration $200/yr
Illinois*	705		396	1,101	No		300	3 yrs	300	Yes	$300 reregistration in state; $600 out of state
Indiana	705		250	955	Yes		250	2 yrs	200	No	
Iowa	760		50	810	Yes		505	2 yrs	450	Yes	Online renewal $450; paper renewal $550
Kansas	705		300	1,005	Yes		400	1 yr	325	Yes	$49 fingerprinting
Kentucky	705		0	705	Yes		300	1 yr	250	Yes	
Louisiana	705		0	705	Yes		382	1 yr	232	Yes	$45.25 fingerprint fee
Maine	705		700	1,405	Yes		450	2 yrs	400	Yes	Added charge for FCVS
Maine DO		675	350	1,025		Yes	350	2 yrs	525	Yes	
Maryland*	705		0	705	Yes		822	2 yrs	518	Yes	
Massachusetts	705		600	1,305	Yes		600	2 yrs	600	Yes	
Michigan	705		150	855	Yes		150	3 yrs	285	Yes	
Michigan DO		675	150	825		Yes	150	3 yrs	285	Yes	
Minnesota	705		200	905	Yes		200	1 yr	192	Yes	
Mississippi	705		600	1,305	Yes		600	1 yr	200	Yes	$200 if renewed online
Missouri	705		300	1,005	No		300	1 yr	135	Yes	
Montana	705		325	1,030	Yes		325	2 yrs	400		
Nebraska	705		300	1,005	Yes		300	2 yrs	121	Yes	

(continued on next page)

Table 15 (continued)
Licensure, Endorsement, and Reregistration Fees, Intervals, and Requirements

	Examination				Application to:			Licensure Reregistration				
	USMLE Step 3 Fee ($)	COMLEX Level 3 Fee ($)	Other Application Fees ($)	Total Cost ($)	FSMB	NBOME	Endorsement Fees ($)	Registration Interval	Regular Fee ($)	CME Credits Required	Notes
Nevada	705		600	1,305	Yes		600	2 yrs	810*	Yes	$75 criminal background investigation fee Reregistration fee $810 online, $850 paper
Nevada DO		675	600	1,275		Yes	600	1 yr	400	Yes	$50 fingerprint fee; FCVS fee additional
New Hampshire	705		250	955	Yes		250	2 yrs	300	Yes	
New Jersey	705		325	1,030	Yes		225	2 yrs	580	Yes	
New Mexico	705		400	1,105	Yes		400	3 yrs	600	Yes	$34 fingerprint fee
New Mexico DO		675	300	975		Yes	300	1 yr	100	Yes	
New York	705		735	1,440	Yes		735	2 yrs	600		
North Carolina*	705		0	705	Yes		350	1 yr	175	Yes	$50 late fee if registration is > 30 days after birthday
North Dakota	705		200	905	Yes		200	1 yr	150	Yes	$450 late fee
Ohio*	705		335*	1,040	Yes	Yes	335*	2 yrs	305	Yes	* FCVS fee additional
Oklahoma	705		400	1,105	Yes		400	1 yr	150	Yes	
Oklahoma DO		675	0	675		Yes		1 yr	225	Yes	$150 late fee
Oregon	705		375	1,080	Yes		375	2 yrs	438	Yes	$150 late fee
Pennsylvania	705		35	740	Yes			2 yrs	360	Yes	
Pennsylvania DO		675	215	890		Yes	45	2 yrs	440	Yes	
Puerto Rico	705		0	705	No		200	3 yrs	75	Yes	
Rhode Island	705		570	1,275	Yes		570	2 yrs	650	Yes	$140 CSR fee
South Carolina	705		0	705	Yes		600	2 yrs	180	Yes	
South Dakota	860		200	1,060	Yes		200	1 yr	200		$400 late fee ($200 reinstatement plus $200 renewal)
Tennessee	705		400	1,105	Yes		235	2 yrs	235	Yes	$280 out-of-state and international application processing fee (nonrefundable)
Tennessee DO		675	400	1,075		Yes		2 yrs	285	Yes	
Texas*	705		885	1,590	Yes			2 yrs	752	Yes	
Utah	705		200	905	Yes		200	2 yrs	183	Yes	$20 late fee; $50 reinstatement fee (FCVS required)
Utah DO		675	200	875		Yes	200	2 yrs	183	Yes	See note above
Vermont	745		2,000	2,745	Yes		625	2 yrs	500		$25 (+ $5/month) late fee
Vermont DO		675	500	1,175		Yes	500	2 yrs	500	Yes	
Virgin Islands	NA	NA	NA	NA	NA		NA	1 yr	500	Yes	
Virginia	705		0	705	Yes		302	2 yrs	337	Yes	
Washington*	705		425	1,130	Yes		425	2 yrs	525	Yes	
Washington DO		675	825	1,500		Yes	825	1 yr	800	Yes	Add $25 for substance abuse monitoring prgm

(continued on next page)

Table 15 (continued)
Licensure, Endorsement, and Reregistration Fees, Intervals, and Requirements

	Examination							Licensure Reregistration			
	USMLE Step 3 Fee ($)	COMLEX Level 3 Fee ($)	Other Application Fees ($)	Total Cost ($)	Application to:		Endorsement Fees ($)	Registration Interval	Regular Fee ($)	CME Credits Required	Notes
					FSMB	NBOME					
West Virginia	705		600	1,305	Yes		300	2 yrs	300	Yes	
West Virginia DO		675	200	875		Yes	200	2 yrs	200	Yes	
Wisconsin*	705		110	815	No		110	2 yrs	106	Yes	Initial $15 contract fee for USMLE Exam
Wyoming	705		450	1,155	Yes		600	1 yr	250	Yes	
Total/Average	**705**	**675**	**359**	**1,061**	**47**	**17**	**392**		**359**	**62**	

Abbreviations

CME—continuing medical education

COMLEX—Comprehensive Osteopathic Medical Licensing Examination

CSR—Controlled Substance Registration (Rhode Island)

FCVS—Federation Credentials Verification Service

FSMB—Federation of State Medical Boards

IMG—international medical graduate

NBOME—National Board of Osteopathic Medical Examiners

USMLE—United States Medical Licensing Examination

* Refer to introductory text to this table for more information on this state's regulations.

Note: *All information should be verified with the licensing board; medical licenses are granted to those physicians meeting all state requirements—at the discretion of the board.*

Continuing Medical Education for Licensure Reregistration

Sixty-two boards require continuing medical education (CME) for license reregistration (Table 16). Some states also mandate CME content, such as HIV/AIDS, risk management, or end of life palliative care. In addition, many states also require that a certain percentage of CME be *AMA PRA Category 1 Credit*™ or equivalent. Forty-three states accept the AMA PRA certificate or application as equivalent for purposes of licensure reregistration. Also accepted by some states are certificates/awards of the American Osteopathic Association (15), American Board of Medical Specialties (27), a state medical society (11), and a national specialty society (6) as well as completion of graduate medical education residency/fellowship programs (34).

Additional Notes for Specific Licensing Jurisdictions

California MD and DO—All general internists and family physicians who have a patient population of which more than 25% are 65 years of age or older shall complete at least 20 hours of all mandatory CME in geriatric medicine or the care of older patients.

All physicians and surgeons (except pathologists and radiologists) must complete mandatory CME in the subjects of pain management and the treatment of terminally ill and dying patients (one-time requirement of 12 credits). Physicians must complete this requirement by their second license renewal date or within 4 years, whichever comes first.

Florida MD—*First time license renewal:* One hour HIV/AIDS, 2 hours in prevention of medical errors. *Second and subsequent renewals:* Two hours in prevention of medical errors. *Every third renewal:* Forty hours, including 2 hours in prevention of medical errors and 2 hours in domestic violence CME. *Note:* End-of-life care and palliative care can no longer be completed in lieu of HIV/AIDS or domestic violence courses.

All CME must be *AMA PRA Category 1 Credit*™, except for domestic violence and prevention of medical errors. Domestic violence and prevention of medical errors courses offered by any state or federal government agency or professional association, including any provider of *AMA PRA Category 1 Credit*™, is acceptable.

Florida DO—*First time license renewal:* One hour HIV/AIDS, risk management, Florida laws and rules, controlled substances; 2 hours domestic violence and prevention of medical errors. Of the remaining required hours, at least 20 must be AOA Category 1-A. *Second*

and subsequent renewals: One hour each in risk management, Florida laws and rules, and controlled substances; 2 hours each in domestic violence and prevention of medical errors. *Every third renewal:* 2 hours of domestic violence. *For each license renewal,* of the remaining required hours at least 20 must be AOA Category 1-A; all other hours (including those in the required content categories) can be either *AMA PRA Category 1 Credit*™ or AOA Cateogory 1-A credit.

CME with regard to risk management, Florida laws and rules, controlled substances, and prevention of medical errors must be obtained by completing live, participatory attendance courses.

Maryland—Partial CME credit is offered for ABMS certification, select peer review, serving as an intervenor or monitor on a physician rehabilitation committee or professional committee, and serving as a preceptor for resident physicians or medical students. For first license renewal, the CME requirement is waived, but the licensee must have completed an approved orientation program.

Missouri—The CME license renewal requirement can be met by a) completing 50 hours *AMA PRA Category 1 Credits*™, AOA Category 1-A or 2-A credits, or American Academy of Family Physicians prescribed credits; b) completing 40 hours of *AMA PRA Category 1 Credit*™ or AOA Category 1-A credit if each course, seminar, or activity includes a post-test of the material covered in the 40 CME credits; c) specialty board certification or recertification; or d) participating in an ACGME- or AOA-approved internship or residency program during the reporting period if at least 60 days of the reporting period were spent in the internship or residency.

New Jersey—The six credits for cultural competence are in addition to the 100-hour requirement for physicians licensed prior to 3/24/05; these credits may be included if licensed after this date. For more information, see: *www.njconsumeraffairs.gov/bme/press/cultural.htm.*

For newly licensed physicians, the Board requires attendance at an orientation program; no CME is given for this.

Tennessee MD—Physicians who focus on providing care to persons with intractable pain should refer to item (6)(c) at: *www.painpolicy.wisc.edu/domestic/states/TN/mbreg.pdf*

Washington MD—The board classifies CME into five different categories. A candidate for relicensure may earn all 200 required hours every 4 years in Category 1; a maximum of 80 hours may be earned in any of the other four categories. See: *http://tinyurl.com/6gbd8w*

Table 16
Continuing Medical Education for Licensure Reregistration

	Required Number of CME Credits per Year(s)	Average Credits per Year	AMA PRA Category 1™ or Equivalent AOA, AAFP or ACOG Credits	Certificates/Awards Accepted as Documentation								State-Mandated CME Content/ Additional Notes
				AMA PRA	AMA PRA app.	AOA	ABMS	SMS	NSS	GME	Other	
Alabama	12 1 yr (See note)	12	12				Yes					25 CME credits required for 2011 renewals; rollovers eliminated in 2011
Alaska	50 2 yrs	25	50	Yes			Yes			Yes		
Arizona	40 2 yrs	20		Yes	Yes		Yes			Yes		
Arizona DO	40 2 yrs	20	12 per yr (AOA 1-A)			Yes	Yes			Yes		
Arkansas	20 1 yr	20	not specified	Yes		Yes				Yes		
California*	100 4 yrs	25	100		Yes		Yes	Yes				Pain management, geriatric medicine, end-of-life care (see page 53)
California DO*	150 3 yrs	50	60 (AOA 1-A or B)			Yes*						Pain management, geriatric medicine, end-of-life care (see page 53); AOA cert. accepted when acompanied by AOA activity registration
Colorado	none											
Connecticut	50 2 yrs	25										Infectious disease, risk management, sexual assault, domestic violence
Delaware	40 2 yrs	20	40		Yes							
DC	50 2 yrs	25	50		Yes	Yes				Yes		
Florida*	40 2 yrs	20	40	Yes						Yes		See page 53
Florida DO*	40 2 yrs	20	20 (AOA 1-A)		Yes					Yes		See page 53
Georgia	40 2 yrs	20	40		Yes	Yes				Yes		
Guam	100 2 yrs	50	25		Yes	Yes			Yes		ACEP	2 credits (every 2 yrs) in ethics
Hawaii	40 2 yrs	20	40	Yes		Yes		Yes	Yes	Yes		
Idaho	40 2 yrs	20	40	Yes	Yes	Yes	Yes			Yes		
Illinois	150 3 yrs	50	60	Yes				Yes	Yes	Yes		SMS, NSS if ACCME-accredited
Indiana	none											
Iowa	40 2 yrs	20	40	Yes			Yes (cert and recert)			Yes		Training for identifying and reporting abuse required every 5 yrs for EM, FM, IM, GP, OB/GYN, and Psych, and others who regularly provide primary care to children and adults
Kansas	50 1 yr	50	20	Yes	Yes		Yes	Yes		Yes		
Kentucky	60 3 yrs	20	30	Yes		Yes			Yes	Yes		One-time domestic violence course for primary care physicans; 2 credits HIV/AIDS every 10 yrs; course must be KY-approved
Louisiana	20 1 yr	20	20	Yes								One-time board orientation course
Maine	100 2 yrs	50	40	Yes	Yes		Yes	Yes		Yes		
Maine DO	100 2 yrs	50	40 (AOA 1-A or B)									Specialists may obtain other than AOA Category 1 credit hours
Maryland*	50 2 yrs	25	50		Yes		Yes†					† Partial credit for ABMS
Massachusetts	100 2 yrs	50	40 (AOA 1-A for DOs)	Yes	Yes		Yes	Yes				Study board requirements; risk management
Michigan	150 3 yrs	50	75		Yes							
Michigan DO	150 3 yrs	50	60 (AOA 1-A or B)			Yes				Yes		

(continued on next page)

Table 16 (continued)
Continuing Medical Education for Licensure Reregistration

	Required Number of CME Credits per Year(s)		Average Credits per Year	AMA PRA Category 1™ or Equivalent AOA, AAFP or ACOG Credits	Certificates/Awards Accepted as Documentation								State-Mandated CME Content/ Additional Notes
					AMA PRA	AMA PRA app.	AOA	ABMS	SMS	NSS	GME	Other	
Minnesota	75	3 yrs	25	75	Yes			Yes				MOCOMP	ABMS cert/recert accepted
Mississippi	40	2 yrs	20	40 (DOs: AOA 1-A)		Yes		Yes*			Yes		Initial certification only (not renewal)
Missouri*	50	2 yrs	25	50				Yes			Yes		See page 53
Montana	none												
Nebraska	50	2 yrs	25	50	Yes		Yes						
Nevada	40	2 yrs	20	40		Yes					Yes		Ethics (2 credits), 20 credits in specialty; other 18 credits can be any in Category 1; 4 credits in WMD/ bioterrorism (new applicants only)
Nevada DO	35	1 yr	35	10 (AOA 1-A)	Yes	Yes	Yes						
New Hampshire	100	2 yrs	50	60	Yes			Yes			Yes		Credits reported to NH Med Society
New Jersey*	100	2 yrs	50	40							Yes		Cultural competence
New Mexico	75	3 yrs	25	75	Yes			Yes			Yes		
New Mexico DO	75	3 yrs	25	75	Yes			Yes				USMLE	Active membership in AOA may replace 75 CME credits
New York	none												Infection control, child abuse
North Carolina	150	3 yrs	50	60									
North Dakota	60	3 yrs	20	60	Yes	Yes		Yes				MOCOMP	
Ohio	100	2 yrs	50	40 (DOs: AOA 1-A or B)		Yes	Yes						CME must be OSMA/OOA-certified
Oklahoma	60	3 yrs	20	60	Yes			Yes			Yes†		†50 hrs for each yr of GME
Oklahoma DO	16	1 yr	16	16 (AOA 1-A or B)									1 credit on prescribing controlled substances (every 2 yrs)
Oregon	30	1 yr (by 2011)	30										
Pennsylvania	100	2 yrs	50	20					Yes		Yes		12 credits risk management or patient safety
Pennsylvania DO	100	2 yrs	50	20 (AOA 1-A)					Yes		Yes		12 credits risk management and patient safety
Puerto Rico	60	3 yrs	20	40	Yes								
Rhode Island	40	2 yrs	20	40	Yes	Yes	Yes	Yes	Yes	Yes	Yes		2 credits: universal precautions, bioterrorism, end of life, OSHA, ethics, or pain management
South Carolina	40	2 yrs	20	40				Yes			Yes		75% specialty education (30 credits every 2 yrs)
South Dakota	none												
Tennessee*	40	2 yrs	20	40	Yes								1 credit (every 2 years) in appropriate prescribing
Tennessee DO	40	2 yrs	20	40 (AOA 1-A or 2-A)									See note above
Texas	24	1 yr	24	12 (DOs: AOA 1-A)	Yes			Yes			Yes		Of 12 Category 1 credits, at least 1 in ethics and/or prof. responsibility
Utah	40	2 yrs	20	40							Yes		

(continued on next page)

Table 16 (continued)
Continuing Medical Education for Licensure Reregistration

	Required Number of CME Credits per Year(s)	Average Credits per Year	AMA PRA Category 1™ or Equivalent AOA, AAFP or ACOG Credits	Certificates/Awards Accepted as Documentation								State-Mandated CME Content/ Additional Notes
				AMA PRA	AMA PRA app.	AOA	ABMS	SMS	NSS	GME	Other	
Utah DO	40 2 yrs	20	40							Yes		
Vermont	none											
Vermont DO	30 2 yrs	15		Yes								At least 12 of 30 credits must be osteopathic med education
Virgin Islands	25 1 yr	25	25									
Virginia	60 2 yrs	30	30		Yes					Yes		
Washington*	200 4 yrs	50	Not specified	Yes			Yes	Yes	Yes			
Washington DO	150 3 yrs	50	60 (AOA 1-A or B)	Yes	Yes		Yes	Yes		Yes	(See note)	Also accepted as equivalent: Current certification of CME from medical practice academies and original certification or recertification within 6 yrs by specialty board
West Virginia	50 2 yrs	25	50	Yes								30 credits related to physician's designated specialty; 2 credits (one-time requirement) in end-of-life care, including pain management
West Virginia DO	32 2 yrs	16	16 (AOA 1-A or B)			Yes				Yes		2 credits (one-time requirement) in end-of-life care, including pain management
Wisconsin	30 2 yrs	15	30	Yes								
Wyoming	60 3 yrs	20	60	Yes		Yes	Yes			Yes		
Total	**62**			**30**	**21**	**15**	**27**	**11**	**6**	**34**	**5**	

Abbreviations

ABMS—American Board of Medical Specialties
ACCME—Accreditation Council for Continuing Medical Education
AMA PRA—American Medical Association Physician's Recognition Award
AOA—American Osteopathic Association
AAFP—American Academy of Family Practice
ACEP—American College of Emergency Physicians
ACOG—American College of Obstetricians and Gynecologists
CMA—California Medical Association
CAFP—California Academy of Family Physicians
CME—continuing medical education
EM—emergency medicine
FM—family medicine
GME—graduate medical education
GP—general practice
MOCOMP—Maintenance of Competence Proram, Royal College of Physicians and Surgeons of Canada
NSS—National specialty society
OOA—Ohio Osteopathic Association
OB/GYN—obstetrics-gynecology

OSHA—Occupational Safety and Health Administration
OSMA—Ohio State Medical Association
Psych—psychiatry
SMS—State medical society
USMLE—United States Medical Licensing Examination
WMD—weapons of mass destruction

* Refer to introductory text to this table for more information on this state's regulations.

Note: *All information should be verified with licensing board; medical licenses are granted to those physicians meeting all state requirements—at the discretion of the board.*

Resident/Fellow Physician Licenses

Sixty-five jurisdictions issue educational licenses, permits, certificates, or registration to resident/fellow physicians in graduate medical education (GME) programs, with fees ranging from $0 to $425 per year (Table 17) (The GME program director generally provides a list of residents/fellows and any other required information directly to the licensing jurisdiction.) In 39 of those jurisdictions, residents/fellows must obtain a new permit/license when changing residency/fellowship programs within the state.

Medical boards in 13 states require that prospective residents have passed United States Medical Licensing Examination (USMLE) Step 1 to receive a permit/license. California, Mississippi, North Dakota, Oklahoma, and Utah require passage of Steps 1 and 2.

Eighteen states require that resident/fellow physicians obtain full licensure (not limited or training licenses) at some point in their training (usually after having completed a certain number of years of GME).

Additional Notes for Specific Licensing Jurisdictions

California—Permits are awarded on an individual basis for a maximum of 5 years to noncitizen physicians for postgraduate work in a California medical school.

International medical graduates (IMGs) must submit an application to determine that all core requirements have been met before they may begin training in California.

Illinois—Limited temporary licenses (valid for 6 months) are awarded to persons in non-Illinois residency programs who are accepted for a specific period of time to perform a portion of that program at a clinical residency program in Illinois due to the lack of adequate facilities in their state.

Visiting Resident Permits are issued for 180 days to persons who have been invited or appointed for a specific period of time to perform a portion of that clinical residency program under the supervision of an Illinois-licensed physician in an Illinois patient care clinic or facility affiliated with the out-of-state GME program.

Massachusetts—Limited registration is issued to physicians enrolled in accredited residency programs and physicians enrolled in fellowships at hospitals with accredited residency programs in the area of the applicant's specialty.

Mississippi—Institutional license is issued to first-year residents and IMGs providing health care in state institutions. Applicants are not required to meet all requirements for permanent unrestricted licensure.

Restricted temporary license is issued to physicians enrolled in first year of GME at the University of Mississippi School of Medicine for practice limited to that school.

Addictionology Fellowship License is issued to physicians admitted for treatment in a board-approved drug and/or alcohol addiction treatment program or to physicians enrolled in fellowship of addictionology of the Mississippi State Medical Association Impaired Professionals Program.

Oregon—Limited license granted to fellows for 1 year and renewed for 1 additional year. Limited license for graduate training granted annually until training is completed.

Pennsylvania—Interim limited license (up to 12 consecutive months) is issued to physicians providing medical service other than at the training location of the licensee's accredited GME program.

Graduate license allows for participation for up to 12 consecutive months in GME within the complex of the hospital to which the licensee is assigned and any satellite facility or other training location used in the program.

South Dakota—Resident physicians practicing within the confines of their residency program are not required to obtain a certificate from the board.

A resident physician who wishes to practice on an irregular basis outside their program may apply for a resident certificate if they have completed at least 1 year of GME and remain enrolled in good standing in their program until successful completion. To apply for this certificate, they must meet South Dakota's examination requirements for completion of the entire USMLE within a 7-year period and passing of each step within three attempts. The fee for this certificate is $50.

Table 17
Resident/Fellow Physician Licenses

	Licenses, Permits, Certificates, & Registration	Must Obtain New Permit/License When Changing Residency Programs Within State	Prospective Residents Applying for License Must Have Passed USMLE Step 1	Full licensure required at any point during training?	Notes
Alabama	Yes				Limited license for residency education only.
Alaska	Yes				Residency permits for up to 36 mos to physicians in accredited residency programs in the US.
Arizona	Yes, $50/yr	Yes	Yes		
Arizona DO	Yes	Yes			
Arkansas	Yes				Education license must be renewed annually.
California*	Yes		Yes (and Step 2)	Yes; after 2 yrs (3 yrs for IMGs)	
California DO				Yes; prior to 3rd yr	No CME required.
Colorado	Yes, $10	Yes			Training license valid for duration of program; renews every 3 yrs.
Connecticut	Yes, $0	Yes			
Delaware	Yes, $25	Yes			Training license must be renewed annually.
DC	Yes, $50	Yes	Yes	Yes	
Florida	Yes, $200	Yes			
Florida DO	Yes, $100	Yes			Training registration number (for residents and fellows).
Georgia	Yes, $100				Board must be notified of resident changing program within state.
Guam	Yes	Yes	Yes	Yes; after 3 yrs	
Hawaii	Yes, $75	Yes			
Hawaii DO	Yes, $75				
Idaho	Yes, $10	Yes		Yes (see note)	After 1 yr GME (US/Canadian graduates), 3 yrs GME (IMGs).
Illinois*	Yes	Yes			
Indiana	Yes, $100	Yes	Yes		Resident permit good for 1 yr, may be renewed annually.
Iowa	Yes, $205	Yes			Resident physician license for GME in board-approved pgm under supervision of licensed physician. Issued for full length of pgm.
Kansas	Yes, $50	Yes			
Kentucky	Yes, $75	Yes	Yes		Institutional Practice Limited License or Residency Training License to physicians beyond first yr of GME while still in training.
Louisiana	Yes, $50	Yes			Intern registration for first 12 mos of GME after completing medical school.
Maine	Yes, $100	Yes	Yes		Educational permits for 1 yr in a specific training program, renewable for 7 yrs.
Maine DO	Yes, $200	Yes			Temp. educational permits for 1 yr in a specific training pgm only.
Maryland	Yes, $100	Yes			Registration of med school grads in GME programs.
Massachusetts*	Yes, $100	Yes	Yes	Yes; after 6 yrs	
Michigan	Yes, $170	Yes		Yes; after 6 yrs	Limited annual license for up to 6 yrs for GME, renewable each yr; includes controlled substance license.
Michigan DO	Yes, $170	Yes		Yes; after 6 yrs	Limited annual license for up to 6 yrs for GME; includes controlled substance license.
Minnesota	Yes, $25	Yes			

(continued on next page)

Table 17 (continued)
Resident/Fellow Physician Licenses

	Licenses, Permits, Certificates, & Registration	Must Obtain New Permit/License When Changing Residency Programs Within State	Prospective Residents Applying for License Must Have Passed USMLE Step 1	Full licensure required at any point during training?	Notes
Mississippi*	Yes, $50/$200		Yes (and Step 2)	Yes; after 5 yrs	
Missouri	Yes, $30	Yes			Temporary licenses issued to residents and fellows only.
Montana	Yes, $100/$50				Refer to 37-3-305, Montana Code Annotated.
Nebraska	Yes, $25	Yes		Yes; after 5 yrs	Temporary educational permits for residents.
Nevada	Yes, $425	Yes		Yes (see note)	Limited 1-yr license for clinical residents ($300 initial, $50 renewal, $75 criminal background investigation). Full licensure usually for fellows/chief residents; depends on program needs.
Nevada DO	Yes, $200	Yes			
New Hampshire	Yes, $35	Yes	Yes		
New Jersey	Yes, $50	Yes		Yes; after 5 yrs	Residency training permit required for unlicensed residents in GY2+.
New Mexico	Yes, $10		Yes	Yes; after 8 yrs	
New Mexico DO	Yes, $25				
New York	Yes, $105				Requires limited permit for all medical school graduates except individuals in ACGME- or AOA-accredited residency programs. Requires ECFMG certificate from all IMGs for limited permit.
North Carolina	Yes, $100 (permit); $125 (registration)	Yes			Limited license to resident physicians (ineligible for licensure by endorsement).
North Dakota	Yes, $25		Yes (and Step 2)		Limited license for residents in clinical program, renewable annually.
Ohio	Yes, $75 (initial) $35 (renewal)	Yes		Yes; after 6 yrs	Training certificate or full license mandatory for residents and clinical fellows.
Oklahoma	Yes, $200	Yes	Yes (and Step 2)		
Oklahoma DO	Yes			Yes; after 1 yr	
Oregon*	Yes, $185	Yes			
Pennsylvania*	Yes, $30				Graduate license renewal fee is $15.
Pennsylvania DO	Yes, $30	Yes			Temporary license for GME valid for up to 12 mos; renewal fee $25.
Puerto Rico	Yes				Internship/residency licenses to qualified applicants enrolled in an ACGME-accredited residency program who have successfully completed the first part of the medical board examination (basic sciences) or its equivalent (NBME, FLEX, or USMLE).
Rhode Island	Yes, $40	Yes		Yes; after 5 yrs	Limited medical registration to residents or fellows. Practice limited to the designated institution and must be under the supervision of a staff physician licensed in RI.
South Carolina	Yes, $150	Yes			Limited licenses for residency programs or limited practices renewable on a yearly basis.
South Dakota*					See page 57.
Tennessee	Yes, $25	Yes			
Tennessee DO	Yes, $50				
Texas	Yes, $144	Yes			

(continued on next page)

Table 17 (continued)
Resident/Fellow Physician Licenses

	Licenses, Permits, Certificates, & Registration	Must Obtain New Permit/License When Changing Residency Programs Within State	Prospective Residents Applying for License Must Have Passed USMLE Step 1	Full licensure required at any point during training?	Notes
Utah	Yes, $200		Yes (and Step 2)		
Vermont	Yes, $70				Limited license to residents, fellows, or house officers enrolled in ACGME-accredited residency programs and working under supervision of licensed physician at a state-licensed institution or clinic.
Vermont DO	Yes, $70				
Virgin Islands	Yes				For residents, institutional license only.
Virginia	Yes, $55				Limited license for fellowship and teaching positions. Temporary licenses (renewable annually) to residents and fellows in accredited programs in Virginia.
Washington	Yes, $385				Limited license to physicians in GME and teaching/research at state institutions and city/county health departments.
Washington DO	Yes, $375				Limited licensure for GME only.
West Virginia					
West Virginia DO	Yes, $50				Educational permit valid for 1 yr; must be renewed annually.
Wisconsin	Yes, $10			Yes; after 5 yrs	Temporary educational certificates for residency education after first year.
Wyoming	Yes, $25			Yes; after 1 yr	
Total	**65**	**39**	**13**	**18**	

* Refer to introductory text to this table for more information on this
state's regulations.

Abbreviations

ACGME—Accreditation Council for Graduate Medical Education

AOA—American Osteopathic Association

ECFMG—Educational Commission for Foreign Medical Graduates

FLEX—Federation Licensing Examination

GME—graduate medical education

GY—graduate year

IMGs—international medical graduates

NBME—National Board of Medical Examiners

USMLE—United States Medical Licensing Examination

Note: *All information should be verified with licensing board;
medical licenses are granted to those physicians meeting all
state requirements—at the discretion of the board.*

Resident/Fellow Physician Licenses: Documentation and Verification

Each state has varying requirements as to the documentation sent to teaching hospitals and/or residents/fellows for those physicians who have a limited educational license for the purposes of graduate medical education. Wall certificates, wallet cards, and letters are three commonly used forms of documentation (Table 18).

In addition, most boards maintain archival records of resident/fellow licenses, for varying periods of time, and 52 boards will provide these records to other state boards for licensing/credentialing purposes.

Table 18
Resident/Fellow Physician Licenses: Documentation and Verification

	Documentation that resident/fellow physicians receive with their license information	Verification of the resident/fellow license is provided to other state boards	Length of time resident/fellow license records are maintained
Alabama		Not applicable	
Alaska	Permit only	Yes	
Arizona	Wallet card	Yes	Since 1964
Arizona DO	Wallet card	Yes	5 yrs
Arkansas	Letter and registration card; later a wall certificate	No	
California		No	
California DO	Wall certificate; wallet card	Yes	
Colorado	License	Yes	Indefinitely
Connecticut	None	No	
Delaware	License sent to hospital	Yes	30 yrs
DC	Letter to program; posted on Web	Yes	2 yrs
Florida	Letter	Yes	
Florida DO	Letter to resident/fellow and letter to program	Yes	Indefinitely
Georgia	Wallet card	Yes	Since 2004
Guam	Primary verification	No	
Hawaii	Pocket ID	Yes	10 yrs
Hawaii DO	Pocket ID	Yes	10 yrs
Idaho	Permit only	Yes	Indefinitely
Illinois	Letter to program; printed license with program name	Yes	Indefinitely
Indiana	Wall certificate	Yes	Indefinitely
Iowa	Letter sent to resident and program	Yes	10 yrs
Kansas	Wall certificate, letter	Yes	Indefinitely
Kentucky	Letter	Yes	Indefinitely
Louisiana	Wall certificate, letter, orientation info, DEA info	Yes	
Maine	Wall certificate, to the program	Yes	Indefinitely
Maine DO	Permit to program, posted on Web	Yes	Indefinitely
Maryland		Yes	4 yrs
Massachusetts	Certificate	Yes	Indefinitely
Michigan	License and wallet card	Yes	Indefinitely
Michigan DO	License and wallet card	Yes	Indefinitely
Minnesota	Letter	Yes	Since 1940
Mississippi	Wallet card	Yes	Indefinitely
Missouri	Wall certificate	Yes	Indefinitely
Montana	Temporary license	Yes	Since January 2004
Nebraska	License card and letter	Yes	Indefinitely
Nevada	Wallet card	Yes	Indefinitely
Nevada DO	Certificate	Yes	Indefinitely
New Hampshire	Letter	Yes	

(continued on next page)

Table 18 (continued)
Resident/Fellow Physician Licenses: Documentation and Verification

	Documentation that resident/fellow physicians receive with their license information	Verification of the resident/fellow license is provided to other state boards	Length of time resident/fellow license records are maintained
New Jersey	Training permit to program	Yes (only to confirm that a training permit was issued; no verification of "standing")	
New Mexico	License sent to program	Yes	3 yrs after GME; 80 yrs if permanently licensed in NM
New Mexico DO	Wall certificate, letter, and wallet certificate	Yes	Since 1992
New York		No	
North Carolina	Certificate	Yes	Indefinitely
North Dakota	Letter with informal certificate	Yes	Since 2001
Ohio	letter to the program	Yes	Since 1999
Oklahoma	Wall certificate, wallet card	Yes	Indefinitely
Oklahoma DO	Wall certificate	No	
Oregon	Certificate of registration	Yes	Records on computer since 1984
Pennsylvania	Wallet card, 5x7 certificate sent to program	Yes	
Pennsylvania DO	Training permit/registration to hospital	Yes	
Puerto Rico		No	
Rhode Island		Yes	25 yrs
South Carolina	Wallet card	Yes	Since 2003
South Dakota	—	—	
Tennessee	None	Yes	Indefinitely
Tennessee DO		No	
Texas	Letter to program	Yes	Records on computer since mid-1980s
Utah	Wall certificate (available for purchase)	—	
Vermont	Hardcopy of license	Yes	
Vermont DO		No	
Virgin Islands	—	—	
Virginia	License renewal certificate	Yes	Indefinitely
Washington	Wall certificate to program only	Yes	Indefinitely
Washington DO	Letter	Yes	75 yrs
West Virginia	Resident/training license not issued	—	
West Virginia DO	Letter	No	
Wisconsin	Wall certificate	Yes	Indefinitely
Wyoming	8 1/2 x 11 certificate	Yes	As of July 1, 2006
Total		**52 Yes**	

Abbreviations

GME—graduate medical education

Note: *All information should be verified with licensing board; medical licenses are granted to those physicians meeting all state requirements—at the discretion of the board.*

Noneducational Temporary or Limited Licenses, Permits, Certificates, and Registration

Fifty boards issue noneducational temporary permits, limited and temporary licenses, or other certificates for the practice of medicine, with fees ranging from $0 to $325 (Table 19). The terms for the issuance of such certificates vary, but in general they must be renewed once a year with a stipulated maximum number of renewals allowed (usually 5 years). Often, a board will issue a temporary license or permit valid until the next board meeting, at which a candidate's application will be considered.

Some states permit state institutions to hire unlicensed physicians to work under the supervision of licensed physicians. In many instances, the state departments of mental health and public health that operate these hospitals will not hire physicians who have not had at least 1 year of graduate medical education in an English-speaking hospital. International medical graduates are generally not considered for these positions unless they are in the United States with a permanent resident visa. An unlicensed physician employed by a state hospital is required in most states to register with the state board of medical examiners, which may issue a limited permit to practice within the institution.

Fourteen jurisdictions issue locum tenens permits, with fees ranging from $0 to $475 (Nevada MD board).

Twenty-eight jurisdictions issue inactive licenses (for physicians who want to maintain licensure in that state although they are currently practicing in another state), with fees ranging from $0 to $438 (Oregon).

Twenty-four jurisdictions issue retired physicians' licenses, with fees ranging from $0 to $150 (Kansas), and 15 issue camp licenses.

Table 19
Noneducational Temporary or Limited Licenses, Permits, Certificates, and Registration

	Noneducational Temporary/Limited Licenses, Permits, and Certificates	Locum Tenens Permits	Inactive Licenses	Retired Physicians' Licenses	Camp Licenses	Additional Notes
Alabama	Yes, $175					Limited license for work in penal and mental institutions.
Alaska*	Yes, $145	Yes	Yes, $250	Yes, $100		Retired physician license: $100 one-time fee.
Arizona*	Yes	Yes, $350				
Arizona DO	Yes	Yes, $300				
Arkansas*	Yes, $50					
California			Yes	Yes, $0		
California DO			Yes, $300			Inactive licensee fee is $300 every 2 yrs.
Colorado			Yes, $195			Reinstatement of inactive license $195.
Connecticut	Yes, $150					Temporary permits (valid for 1 yr only, not renewable or extendable) only to those physicians who have been offered a position in a state hospital or state facility.
Delaware						
DC			Yes, $312			
Florida*	Yes (See page 68)		Yes, $55			
Florida DO	Yes, $100		Yes, $100	Yes, $55		
Georgia	Yes, $100		Yes, $140			Temporary permits for endorsement applicants between board meetings.
Guam	Yes, $275		Yes, $300			Temporary permits for reciprocity/endorsement applicants between board meetings.
Hawaii*	Yes					Not available to physicians against whom disciplinary action is pending in another state.
Idaho	Yes, $100		Yes, $75	Yes		Temporary license while awaiting criminal background check outcome; clear routine applicants only; all requirements met; complete application required; good for 120 days. May be extended by board order. Inactive license holders may not practice or prescribe. Volunteer license to retired physicians for uncompensated practice (no fee).
Illinois*	Yes		Yes			
Indiana*	Yes, $100	Yes, $100	Yes, $100	Yes, $100	Yes, $100	
Iowa*	Yes, $155					
Kansas*	Yes, $30		Yes, $150	Yes, $150		Physicians with inactive licenses may not practice medicine in any form, including writing prescriptions. Limited to charity work.
Kentucky*	Yes, $75					Temporary permit until board meets (for endorsement candidates only).
Louisiana*	Yes, $0			Yes, $100		
Maine	Yes, $300	Yes		Yes	Yes, $150	Retired physicians' license for those doing volunteer work; volunteer license is $75; temporary and camp licenses (up to 1 yr) for duration of community need.
Maine DO	Yes	Yes, $200			Yes, $100	
Maryland			Yes, $50			Physicians with inactive licenses may not practice medicine in any form, including writing prescriptions. Residents must register with the board annually.

(continued on next page)

Table 19 (continued)
Noneducational Temporary or Limited Licenses, Permits, Certificates, and Registration

	Noneducational Temporary/Limited Licenses, Permits, and Certificates	Locum Tenens Permits	Inactive Licenses	Retired Physicians' Licenses	Camp Licenses	Additional Notes
Massachusetts		Yes				
Michigan				Yes, $0		For practice in underserved areas, with no remuneration; reviewed annually.
Michigan DO				Yes, $0		For practice in underserved areas, with no remuneration; reviewed annually.
Minnesota	Yes, $60			Yes, $50	Yes, $0	Temporary license valid until next board meeting at which application is to be considered.
Mississippi	Yes				Yes, $25	Ninety-day Youth Camp Permit issued to physicians providing health care only at youth camps approved by the Mississippi State Department of Health.
Missouri				Yes, $25	Yes	Camp license not required if service is less than 2 weeks.
Montana	Yes, $325		Yes	Yes		
Nebraska*		Yes, $100	Yes, $35			
Nevada	Yes	Yes, $475	Yes, $400			Locum tenens license (not renewable) for 90 days to qualified candidates. Temporary licenses for practice in medically underserved areas (at discretion of the board). $75 criminal background investigation fee.
Nevada DO	Yes, $200		Yes, $200			
New Hampshire*	Yes, $150	Yes, $150			Yes, $75	
New Jersey*	Yes			Yes, $125		
New Mexico	Yes, $100		Yes, $25		Yes, $50	
New Mexico DO	Yes, $0					Issued to physicians who have applied for and met licensure requirements between regular board meetings.
New York	Yes					Retired physicians exempt from registration fee.
North Carolina	Yes, $150			Yes, $0; registration is $25	Yes, $100	Limited license for practice in medically underserved areas; retired volunteer license and military volunteer for indigent clinics and summer camps only.
North Dakota*	Yes, $200	Yes, $200		Yes		Locum tenens permit not to exceed 3 months; no fee for lifetime special emeritus license status (may not practice).
Ohio*	Yes		Yes, $0 volunteer certificate	Yes, $0 Emeritus certificate		Limited certificates for employment in state hospitals. Retired physician license. Special activity certificate $125.
Oklahoma*	Yes			Yes		Emeritus (may not practice); limited volunteer license for uncompensated practice.
Oklahoma DO				Yes		Emeritus (may not practice); limited volunteer license for uncompensated practice.
Oregon*	Yes, $185		Yes, $438		Yes, $438	Locum tenens license limited to 240 days' practice in state in the biennium, limited license, SPEX.
Pennsylvania*	Yes			Yes		
Pennsylvania DO	Yes			Yes	Yes, $45	
Puerto Rico*	Yes					
Rhode Island			Yes, $0			Emeritus status (inactive license).
South Carolina	Yes, $75		Yes, $0			Temporary license to any applicant who meets all requirements pending final board approval.

(continued on next page)

Table 19 (continued)
Noneducational Temporary or Limited Licenses, Permits, Certificates, and Registration

	Noneducational Temporary/Limited Licenses, Permits, and Certificates	Locum Tenens Permits	Inactive Licenses	Retired Physicians' Licenses	Camp Licenses	Additional Notes
South Dakota		Yes, $50				Sixty-day locum tenens permit.
Tennessee	Yes	Yes				
Tennessee DO						
Texas*	Yes, $50			Yes		Temporary licenses pending final board approval.
Utah			Yes, $50			Inactive license must be renewed every 2 yrs; $50 to make active again.
Vermont						
Vermont DO	Yes					
Virgin Islands	Yes					Temp licenses (2 yrs) for government employment only.
Virginia	Yes		Yes, $168		Exemption authorized $25	Exemptions authorized for continuing education, summer camps, and free clinics. Volunteer restricted license issued for practice in free clinics.
Washington	Yes, $50			Yes		Temporary permit (valid 90 days) only in conjunction with full application; applicant must have been previously licensed in an approved state.
Washington DO	Yes		Yes			Must be applicant for a full license; valid for 90 days. Not renewable. Must be licensed and in good standing in another state.
West Virginia	Yes, $100		Yes, $100		Yes	If eligible, temporary license (valid until subsequent board meeting) is issued, after completed application for permanent license has been filed, processed, and found in order.
West Virginia DO	Yes					Temporary license granted, at discretion of board, for specific location and need.
Wisconsin	Yes	Yes, $163			Yes, $163	Camp physician license or locum tenens for up to 90 days.
Wyoming	Yes, $200		Yes; only if living in state	Yes; only if living in state	Yes	Temporary license between board meetings after completed application for permanent license has been filed, processed, and approved by the board.
Total	**50**	**14**	**28**	**24**	**15**	

* Refer to additional text on following pages for more information on this state's regulations.

Abbreviations

GME—graduate medical education

SPEX—Special Purpose Examination

USMLE—United States Medical Licensing Examination

Note: *All information should be verified with licensing board; medical licenses are granted to those physicians meeting all state requirements—at the discretion of the board.*

(continued on next page)

Table 19 (continued)
Noneducational Temporary or Limited Licenses, Permits, Certificates, and Registration

Alaska
- Temporary permits for specific period (6 months maximum) after completed application is on file and until board meets to consider permanent licensure.
- Locum tenens permit for 90 days to an MD or DO licensed in another state for purpose of substituting for another Alaska-licensed physician; may extend 1-60 days.

Arizona
- Locum tenens permit for a 180-day period to a licensed MD to temporarily assist or substitute for an MD licensed in Arizona.

Arkansas
- Temporary permits for limited time in emergency or hardship cases, only after application for licensure is complete and waiting to be presented to the board. Valid until next board meeting.

Florida
- Temporary Certificate to Practice in Area of Critical Need ($300) to MDs/DOs with current valid license in another state to practice in Florida communities with a critical need for physicians and a population of less than 7,500.
- Limited License ($210) to MDs/DOs who meet the same minimum education and training requirements as required for a full medical license and who are retired and have been licensed to practice medicine in any jurisdiction in the United States for at least 10 yrs. Practice restricted to public agencies or institutions or nonprofit agencies or institutions meeting the requirements of Section 501(c)(3) of the Internal Revenue Code and located in areas of critical medical need.
- A Public Psychiatry Certificate to board-certified psychiatrists who are licensed to practice medicine without restriction in another state and who meet the minimum education and training requirements required for a full medical license. Practice is restricted to a public mental health facility or program funded in part or entirely by state funds.
- A Public Health Certificate to MDs/DOs who are graduates of an accredited medical/osteopathic school and hold a master of public health degree or are board-eligible or certified in public health or preventive medicine, or to MDs/DOs who are licensed to practice medicine without restriction in another jurisdiction in the United States and hold a master of public health degree or are board eligible or certified in public health or preventive medicine and who meet the minimum education and training requirements required for a full medical/osteopathic license. Practice restricted to employment duties with the Department of Health and Rehabilitative Services.

Hawaii
- Temporary license to physicians working in a state or county agency in conditions of shortage or emergency; and to physicians under the supervision of a licensed MD who plan to take the USMLE exam within 18 months.

Illinois
- Visiting Physician Permits for up to 180 days to persons receiving an invitation or appointment to study, demonstrate, or perform a specific medical, osteopathic, or chiropractic subject or technique in medical, osteopathic, or chiropractic schools; hospitals; or facilities operated pursuant to the Ambulatory Surgical Treatment Center Act.

Indiana
- To physicians holding an active, valid license from another US/Canadian jurisdiction who have applied for and are awaiting board approval of permanent unrestricted license by endorsement of another jurisdiction's valid license; valid for a designated period of 90 days or less.
- To physicians holding a valid, active license from another US/Canadian jurisdiction who are providing health care for a circumscribed period as part of a special program, event, or other activity, including locum tenens; permit valid for up to 30 days and is not renewable.

Iowa
Temporary licensure is intended for physicians to participate in any of the following board-approved activities:

- Covering for an Iowa licensed physician who unexpectedly is unavailable to provide medical care to the physician's patients
- Demonstrating or proctoring that involves providing hands on patient care to patients in Iowa
- Conducting a procedure on a patient in Iowa when the consultant's expertise in the procedure is greater than that of the Iowa licensed physician who requested the procedure
- Providing medical care to patients in Iowa, if the physician is enrolled in an out-of-state GME program and does not hold a resident or permanent license in the home state of the GME program
- Serving as a camp physician
- Participating as a learner in a program of further medical education that allows hands-on patient care when the physician does not currently hold a license in good standing in any US jurisdiction
- Any other activity approved by the board

Temporary licensure is not to be used as a way for a physician to practice before a permanent license is granted. It is also not intended for locum tenens.

Kansas
- Out-of-phase special permit.
- Limited license for charity work if licensee is in another state.

Kentucky
- Temporary permit until next licensure board meeting after application for licensure has been completed, filed, processed, and found to be in order. No temporary permit before passing examination.

Louisiana
- Unrestricted temporary permits only under extreme circumstances. Board meets every 4 weeks to act on reciprocity licensure applications. Board must act on SPEX applicants requiring unrestricted temporary permit. SPEX applicants issued institutional temporary permit, if necessary, pending results of exam.
- Ninety-day renewable unrestricted permit, pending valid visa issued by the Immigration and Naturalization Service.

(continued on next page)

Table 19 (continued)
Noneducational Temporary or Limited Licenses, Permits, Certificates, and Registration

Nebraska	• Locum tenens permit for a qualified physician with current license in another state for replacement of a Nebraska physician during a period of temporary leave (maximum of 90 days in any 12-month period).
New Hampshire	• Temporary/restricted license, in the state's best interest. Locum tenens (courtesy license) available to a qualified applicant currently holding an unrestricted active license in another state; valid for a maximum of 100 consecutive days in any 12-month period.
New Jersey	• Temporary license (4 months) for a lawfully qualified physician of another state to take charge of the practice of a licensed New Jersey physician during his or her absence from the state. Exemption from licensure to work in county or state institution for a limited period.
North Dakota	• Temporary license between intervals of board meetings; permanent licenses issued only at regularly scheduled meetings (March, July, and November). All licensure requirements must be met and file must be processed completely before a temporary license or locum tenens permit will be issued.
Ohio	• Special Activity Certificate ($125) may be issued to qualified applicants seeking to practice in conjunction with a special activity, program, or event taking place in Ohio. The certificate may not be used for locum tenens, is valid for the shorter of 30 days or the duration of the special activity, and cannot be renewed.
Oklahoma	• Temporary medical licenses during the intervals between board meetings. Candidates for temporary license must meet qualifications for full and unrestricted license. Temporary licenses automatically terminate on the date of the next board meeting, when the applicant may be considered for a full and unrestricted medical license.

Oregon	• Limited License SPEX (LL-SPEX) valid while awaiting results of SPEX examination.
Pennsylvania	• Temporary License allows licensee to participate in a medical procedure necessary for the well-being of a specified patient within the Commonwealth or to practice medicine and surgery at a camp or resort for no more than 3 months. Applicants for a temporary license must hold an unrestricted license in another state, territory, possession, or country.
	• Extraterritorial License granted to licensed physicians maintaining an office to practice near the boundary line of an adjoining state whose medical practice extends into Pennsylvania.
Puerto Rico	• Public service licenses to qualified applicants who have completed at least 1 yr of accredited residency education and who have passed all three parts of the medical board examination or its equivalent (NBME, FLEX, or USMLE).
Texas	• Telemedicine • Public Health • Conceded Eminence • Faculty Temporary License • Voluntary Charity Care

Note: *All information should be verified with the licensing board; medical licenses are granted to those physicians meeting all state requirements—at the discretion of the board.*

Physician Reentry

The AMA defines physician reentry as "a return to clinical practice in the discipline in which one has been trained or certified following an extended period of clinical inactivity not resulting from discipline or impairment." Twenty-nine states have specific rules for physicians seeking to reenter clinical practice, such as requiring passage of the Special Purpose Examination (SPEX) (see page 98), and nine states are in the process of developing such policy; others review physicians in this category on a case-by-case basis (Table 20).

The Physician Reentry into the Workforce Project

The issue of physician reentry into the workforce after a period of clinical and/or professional inactivity (not resulting from discipline or impairment) is growing in importance. Anecdotal evidence indicates that reentry into the workforce will affect women more often than men (and the numbers of women entering medical school continue to grow), but this is an issue that cuts across genders and specialties.

To address this growing concern, a number of organizations and individuals are participating in a collaborative endeavor, The Physician Reentry into the Workforce Project, to examine reentry and create guidelines, recommendations, and strategies that will serve to assist physicians and protect patients.

Managed by the American Academy of Pediatrics, Division of Workforce and Medical Education Policy, project participants include representatives of:

- Accreditation Council for Continuing Medical Education
- American Medical Association:
  - Medical Education Group
  - Women Physicians' Congress
- American Academy of Family Physicians
- American Academy of Pediatrics, Committee on Pediatric Education
- American Board of Medical Specialties
- American College of Physicians
- American Osteopathic Association
- Association of American Medical Colleges
- Council on Graduate Medical Education
- Council on Medical Specialty Societies
- Drexel University College of Medicine REMED Program
- Federation of State Medical Boards
- National Board of Medical Examiners
- Naval Medical Center San Diego
- Northeastern Ohio Universities Colleges of Medicine & Pharmacy
- The Joint Commission
- University of California-San Diego Physician Assessment & Clinical Education (PACE) Program

Four topic-specific workgroups have been established to advance the project's agenda:

- Assessment and Evaluation
- Education
- Credentialing, Licensure, and Maintenance of Certification
- Workforce

The Credentialing, Licensure and Maintenance of Certification Workgroup is seeking to identify strategies to help physicians maintain their professional standing while they are absent from the workforce. It will also propose a process for physicians to regain their professional credentials if they lose them and wish to return to active clinical practice. This workgroup's key issues, challenges, and opportunities include:

- Obtaining knowledge regarding the policies of licensing, certifying, and credentialing bodies and staying current with evolving standards and requirements for physicians from various regulatory agencies

- Exploring the need for pertinent regulatory agencies to define reentry policies for their constituents

- Identifying what types of policies regulatory agencies and boards should have regarding how to best communicate their reentry requirements to those licensed in their jurisdiction

- Identifying the challenges for physicians who choose to leave the workforce in the areas of licensure, board certification, and hospital privileges and identifying barriers to reentry that regulatory agencies may impose, even inadvertently.

- Identifying strategies to help physicians maintain their professional standing while they are absent from the physician workforce.

- Identifying current programs that assist physicians in regaining their professional credentials

- Proposing a process for physicians to regain their professional credentials if they lose them and wish to return to clinical practice

- Identifying current programs that assist physicians in regaining their professional credentials

Current members of this workgroup are:

- Carol Clothier, Co-Chair
  Federation of State Medical Boards

- Richard E. Hawkins, MD, Co-Chair
  National Board of Medical Examiners

- Elizabeth A. Bower, MD, MPH
  Oregon Health Sciences University

- Frank Dornfest, MB, ChB, MFGP (SA), FAAFP
  Oregon Health Sciences University

- Sheldon D. Horowitz, MD, FAAP
  American Board of Medical Specialties

- Saralyn Mark, MD, Content Expert
  SolaMed Solutions, LLC

- Lawrence Nazarian, MD, FAAP
  American Academy of Pediatrics,
  Committee on Pediatric Education

- Paul M. Schyve, MD
  The Joint Commission

- Melissa Thomas, MD, PhD
  Laboratory of Molecular Endocrinology,
  Massachusetts General Hospital

- Kelly J. Towey, MEd
  Reentry Project Consultant

Contact information

Physician Reentry into the Workforce Project
American Academy of Pediatrics, Division of Workforce and Medical Education Policy
141 Northwest Point Boulevard
Elk Grove Village, IL 60007-1098
(847) 434-4000
(847) 434-8000 Fax

Holly J. Mulvey, MA, Reentry Project Co-Director
E-mail: *hmulvey@aap.org*

Diamond Lanier, Department Assistant
E-mail: *dlanier@aap.org*

Web site

In addition to serving as a forum for the organizations involved in the project, the Physician Reentry into the Workforce Web site has been enhanced to include resources for individual physicians seeking reentry information.

www.aap.org/reentry

AMA Council on Medical Education Report on Physician Reentry

At its 2008 annual meeting, the AMA House of Delegates adopted as AMA policy the recommendations of AMA Council on Medical Education Report 6, Physician Reentry, asking that the AMA:

1. Continue to collaborate with other appropriate organizations on physician reentry issues including research on the need for and the effectiveness of reentry programs.

2. Work collaboratively with the American Academy of Pediatrics and other interested groups to convene a conference on physician reentry which will bring together key stakeholders to address the development of reentry programs as well as the educational needs of physicians reentering clinical practice.

3. Work with interested parties to establish a physician reentry program information data base that is publicly accessible to physician applicants and which includes information pertaining to program characteristics.

4. Support efforts to ensure the affordability and accessibility, and to address the unique liability issues related to physician reentry programs.

5. Make available to all interested parties the physician reentry program system Guiding Principles for use as a basis for all reentry programs:

a. *Accessible: The reentry program system is accessible by geography, time, and cost.* Reentry programs are available and accessible geographically across the United States and include national and regional pools of reentry positions. Reentering physicians with families or community ties are not burdened by having to relocate to attend a program. The length of time of reentry programs is standardized and is commensurate with the assessed clinical and educational needs of reentering physicians. The cost of reentry programs is not prohibitive to the physician, health care institutions, or the health care system.

b. *Collaborative: The reentry program system is designed to be collaborative to improve communication and resource sharing.* Information and materials including evaluation instruments are shared across specialties, to the extent possible, to improve program and physician performance. A common nomenclature is used to maximize communication across specialties. Reentry programs share resources and create a common repository for such resources, which are easily accessible.

c. *Comprehensive: The reentry program system is comprehensive to maximize program utility.* Physician reentry programs prepare physicians to return to clinical activity in the discipline in which they have been trained or certified and in the practice settings they expect to work including community-based, public health, and hospital-based or academic practice.

d. *Ethical: The reentry program system is based on accepted principles of medical ethics.* Physician reentry programs will conform to physician licensure statues. The standards of professionalism, as stated in the AMA Code of Medical Ethics, must be followed.

e. *Flexible: The reentry program system is flexible in structure in order to maximize program relevancy and usefulness.* Physician reentry programs can accommodate modifications to program requirements and activities in ways that are optimal to the needs of reentering physicians.

f. *Modular: Physician reentry programs are modularized, individualized, and competency-based.* They are tailored to the learning needs of reentering physicians, which prevents the need for large, expensive, and standardized programs. Physicians should only be required to take those modules that allow them to meet an identified educational need.

g. *Innovative: Innovation is built into a reentry program system, allowing programs to offer state of the art learning and meet the diverse and changing needs of reentry physicians.* Physician reentry programs develop and utilize learning tools including experimenting with innovative and novel curricular methodologies such as distance learning technologies and simulation.

h. *Accountable: The reentry program system has mechanisms for assessment and is open to evaluation.* Physician reentry programs have an evaluation component that is comparable among all specialties. Program assessments use objective measures to evaluate physician's competence at time of entry, during the program, and at time of completion. Program outcomes are measured. Reliability and validity of the measures are established. Standardization of measures exist across programs to assess whether or not national standards are being met.

i. *Stable: A funding scheme is in place to ensure the reentry program system is financially stable over the long-term.* Adequate funding allows physician reentry programs to operate at sufficient and appropriate capacity.

j. *Responsive: The reentry program system makes refinements, updates, and other changes when necessary.* Physician reentry programs are equipped to address systemic changes such as changes in regulations. Additionally, the reentry program system is prepared to respond efficiently to urgent health care needs within society including mobilizing clinically inactive physicians temporarily into the workforce to attend to an acute public health crisis, such as a terrorist, biological, chemical, or natural disaster.

6. As part of its Initiative to Transform Medical Education strategic focus and in support of its members and Federation partners, develop model program standards utilizing physician reentry program system Guiding Principles with a report back at the 2009 Interim Meeting.

AMA Initiative to Transform Medical Education (ITME) and Physician Reentry

Since its inception in 2005, the AMA Initiative to Transform Medical Education (ITME) has identified opportunities for improvement in physician education (Phase 1) and developed general recommendations for change across the medical education continuum (Phase 2). A report summarizing Phase 1 and 2 outcomes is available on the AMA Council on Medical Education Web site at *www.ama-assn.org/go/councilmeded*

Currently, ITME is in the third of its three phases, focusing on conducting in-depth research and planning for change in a number of priority areas. In addition to the medical education learning environment, medical school admissions, and physician self-assessment and lifelong learning, ITME's priority list now includes the topic of physician reentry to practice, due to the relative scarcity of and increasing need for reentry programs. To that end, ITME has recommended that the medical education system "consider creating alternatives to the current sequence of the medical education continuum, including introducing options so that physicians can reenter or modify their practices."

Since its inception, ITME has espoused the idea that collaboration and the participation of a wide variety of relevant stakeholders in the health care community is critical to successful outcomes. This is especially true for efforts related to physician reentry. As an example of this collaboration, the AMA and the American Academy of Pediatrics cosponsored the Physician Reentry into the Workforce conference in September 2008, bringing together experts and stakeholders who identified and prioritized plans for future work in four areas:

- Workforce implications
- Regulatory issues, such as licensure
- Assessment and evaluation of competence
- Design and content of reentry programs

Participants generated a variety of suggestions for future data gathering and implementation activities, ranging from developing plans for continuing medical education and career planning activities to disseminating information about existing reentry programs to those who seek to return to the workforce.

Contact Information

AMA Council on Medical Education
515 N State St
Chicago, IL 60654
www.ama-assn.org/go/councilmeded

Table 20
Physician Reentry Regulations

	Board has policy on physician reentry to practice*	Length of time out of practice after which reentry program completion is required	Board developing/ planning to develop policy	Notes
Alabama	No		No	
Alaska	No		Yes	
Arizona	No		No	
Arizona DO	No		Yes	
Arkansas	No		No	
California	No			Board is not permitted to request of a licensee whether the licensee is in active clinical practice. If license is placed in an inactive status, physician must pay fees and complete CME to reactivate; if license canceled, must completely reapply for licensure.
California DO	Yes	5 yrs	—	Must complete a questionnaire provided by Board; submit CME documentation completed within 12 months of reentry, and pay fees. To activate an inactive license, physician must pay fees and complete CME. If license is cancelled, physician must reapply for new license.
Colorado	Yes	2 yrs	—	Personalized competency evaluation report prepared by a Board-approved program, and completion of any education/training recommended by the program as a result of the evaluation. Complete reentry education program upon reactivation or reinstatement or for new applicant.
Connecticut	No			
Delaware	No		No	
DC	No		Yes	Physicians not actively practicing for 1 to 5 yrs must submit proof of 50 Category 1 CME credits for each inactive year. To reactivate a paid inactive license after 5 yrs, either 1 yr of clinical training in an ACGME- or AOA-accredited program or 300 Category 1 CME credits is required.
Florida	Yes	2 yrs for inactive, 5 yrs for retired	—	Physicians with a retired status license who have not practiced in another jurisdiction for 5 or more yrs must pass SPEX; those with an inactive status license who have not practiced in another jurisdiction for 2 of the previous 4 yrs must pass SPEX.
Florida DO	Yes	5 yrs	—	Board recommends Univ. of Florida CARES or CAPS program.
Georgia	Yes	2 yrs	—	If over 2 yrs, a physician must be able to demonstrate current knowledge, skill, and proficiency.
Guam				
Hawaii	No		No	
Hawaii DO				
Idaho	No		No	
Illinois	Yes	2 yrs	—	Detailed information is in Section 1285.95 of the Administrative Rules.
Indiana	No		No	Physicians who let their licenses lapse for more than 3 yrs and are reapplying are reviewed on a case-by-case basis; personal appearance before the Board is required.
Iowa	Yes	3 yrs	—	If physician is applying for a permanent license or reinstating an inactive license to active status and has not practiced within the past 3 yrs in the US/Canada, a competency evaluation is required.
Kansas	Yes	2 yrs	—	Disciplinary plan to adhere to requirements.
Kentucky	No		No	
Louisiana	Yes		—	Applicant would have to meet the requirements for reinstatement or relicensure. Additional information at www.lsbme.la.gov.
Maine	Yes	Over 1 yr		Depends on the situation.
Maine DO	No		No	
Maryland	Yes	Case by case	—	Determined on a case-by-case basis. Passing SPEX may be required. A physician whose license has been placed on inactive status or who has failed to renew a license by the 2-month late renewal period and who wishes to practice medicine in Maryland may apply for reinstatement.

(continued on next page)

Table 20 (continued)
Physician Reentry Regulations

	Board has policy on physician reentry to practice*	Length of time out of practice after which reentry program completion is required	Board developing/ planning to develop policy	Notes
Massachusetts	No	Yes		Board requires physician to present a practice plan for reentry to practice if not engaged in direct patient care for more than 2 yrs.
Michigan	No		No	
Michigan DO	No		No	Complete 150 hours of CME with a minimum of 60 hrs in AOA Category 1 activities within immediately previous 3 yrs from date of application.
Minnesota	Yes	2-3 yrs	—	Board reviews on case-by-case basis; generally includes assessment, CME, mentorship, SPEX.
Mississippi	Yes	3 yrs	—	Complete a Board-approved physician assessment or clinical skills assessment program.
Missouri	Yes	2 yrs	—	
Montana	Yes	2 yrs	—	SPEX required if applicant not engaged in the active practice of medicine for 2 or more yrs.
Nebraska	No		—	Board reviews on case-by-case basis.
Nevada	Yes	1 yr	—	Full Board appearance, possibility of peer review or another exam to prove competence.
Nevada DO	Yes		—	Requires proof of CME for all yrs a physician is not licensed with the Board. Inactive status $200 per yr. Additional $200 and proof of CME for inactive yrs required to reactivate practice.
New Hampshire	No		No	No formal policy; decided on case-by-case basis.
New Jersey	Yes	5 yrs	—	
New Mexico	Yes	Over 2 yrs	—	Mini-Sabbatical or participation in CPEP's Clinical Practice Re-Entry Program may be required.
New Mexico DO				
New York	No		No	A licensed physician in inactive status must re-register. If new practice requirements have been enacted, physicians must meet these requirements.
North Carolina	Yes	2 yrs	—	Completion of reentry program required.
North Dakota	No		No	Addressed on case-by-case basis; a reentry plan is developed as appropriate.
Ohio	Yes	2 yrs	—	Board may require an applicant for licensure restoration to pass an exam to determine current fitness to practice. SPEX or Board certification/recertification examination may be required.
Oklahoma	No		Yes	
Oklahoma DO	No			Decided on case-by-case basis.
Oregon	Yes	2 yrs (may differ based on specialty)	—	A physician out of practice more than 12 months may be required to take a competency exam or training.
Pennsylvania	Yes	4 yrs	—	Requirements include CME and, depending on length of time out of practice, reentry to practice plan, including any of the following: successful completion of a clinical skills assessment program, refresher training, mentorship program, a mini-residency, passage of SPEX exam, passage of ABMS board exams, etc.
Pennsylvania DO	No		Yes	Additional training or SPEX may be required, as well as completion of application, proof of CME, and payment of fee.
Puerto Rico				
Rhode Island	No		Yes	Decided on a case-by-case basis and often including specific requirements such as mentorship or CME. Reactivation or reapplication, depending on amount of time lapsed and reason.
South Carolina	No		No	

(continued on next page)

Table 20 (continued)
Physician Reentry Regulations

	Board has policy on physician reentry to practice*	Length of time out of practice after which reentry program completion is required	Board developing/ planning to develop policy	Notes
South Dakota	No		Yes	No formal policy, Board discretion.
Tennessee	Yes	5 yrs	—	Determined on case-by-case basis. Must display clinical competency.
Tennessee DO	Yes	5 yrs	—	Determined on case-by-case basis. Must display clinical competency.
Texas	Yes		—	Board reentry policy does not apply to physicians already licensed who are renewing. Must have been in active practice for one of the 2 yrs preceding the date of application for licensure in Texas.
Utah	Yes	2 yrs	—	SPEX may be required.
Vermont	No	5 yrs	Yes	SPEX may be required.
Vermont DO	Yes	1 yr	—	SPEX may be required.
Virgin Islands				
Virginia	Yes	4 yrs	—	SPEX exam may be required if a physician has not practiced in over 4 yrs.
Washington	Yes	2 yrs	—	SPEX exam, or any other examination deemed appropriate, may be required.
Washington DO	No		No	
West Virginia	No	18 months	No	
West Virginia DO	No		No	
Wisconsin	No	5 yrs	No	After 5 yrs, full reapplication is required; all application questions must be answered and oral examination may be required. If less than 5 yrs, renewal is allowed. Re-registration application is required ($188).
Wyoming	No		Yes	Determined on case-by-case basis; SPEX or other display of clinical competence may be required.
Total (Yes)	**29**		**9**	

* As defined by the AMA

Abbreviations
ACGME—Accreditation Council for Graduate Medical Education
ABMS—American Board of Medical Specialties
AOA—American Osteopathic Association
CME—continuing medical education
CPEP—Center for Personalized Education for Physicians
SPEX—Special Purpose Examination

Note: *All information should be verified with licensing board; medical licenses are granted to those physicians meeting all state requirements—at the discretion of the board.*

Regulations on the Practice of Telemedicine and Out-of-state Consulting Physicians

For purposes of this publication, *telemedicine* is defined as the delivery of health care services via electronic means from a health care provider in one location to a patient in another. Applications that fall under this definition include the transfer of medical images, such as pathology slides or radiographs, interactive video consultations between patient and provider or between primary care and specialty care physicians, and mental health consultations. A number of states have adopted or have begun to develop regulations concerning the practice of telemedicine (Table 21).

The AMA has monitored the development of telemedicine over the years and has official policy on this issue (see Appendix E, AMA Policy on Medical Licensure). At its 2008 annual meeting, for example, the AMA House of Delegates adopted resolution 317, proposed by the AMA Resident and Fellow Section, asking that the AMA work with the Federation of State Medical Boards "to study how guidelines regulating medical licenses are affected by telemedicine and medical technological innovations that allow for physicians to practice outside their states of licensure."

Physician Licensure During Emergency Situations and Disasters

In addition to telemedicine and out-of-state consultation in day-to-day practice, the issue of licensing out-of-state volunteer physicians during emergency situations and disasters is increasing in importance.

The results of a 2007 national survey of state medical boards on this topic found that:

- Eighteen (35%) do not permit expedited physician licensure or exemption

- Thirty-two states and the District of Columbia (65%) had statutes specifically granting licensure for volunteer physicians during a disaster

- Thirteen of these 32 states offered licensure via expedited process, while 19 states and the District of Columbia offered licensure through exemption (direct reciprocity)

Source: Lori A. Boyajian-O'Neill; Lindsey M. Gronewold; Alan G. Glaros; Amy M. Elmore. "Physician Licensure During Disasters: A National Survey of State Medical Boards." *JAMA.* 2008;299(2):169-171.

Additional Notes for Specific Licensing Jurisdictions

Mississippi—Full license required for physicians rendering a medical opinion concerning diagnosis or treatment via electronic or other means, unless the evaluation, treatment, and/or medical opinion to be rendered by a physician outside this state (a) is requested by a physician duly licensed to practice medicine in this state, and (b) the physician who has requested such evaluation, treatment, and/or medical opinion has already established a doctor/patient relationship with the patient to be evaluated and/or treated.

Table 21
Regulations on the Practice of Telemedicine and Out-of-state Consulting Physicians

	Practice of Telemedicine		
	Has Adopted Regulations	Has Begun to Develop Regulations	Specific Licensure Restrictions on and/or Requirements for Out-of-state Consulting Physicians
Alabama	Yes		Issues a "special purpose" license (1997).
Alaska			Active Alaska license required. Exceptions are made for an MD or DO who is not a resident of Alaska and who is asked by an Alaskan MD or DO to help in the diagnosis or treatment of a case.
Arizona	Yes		No license required for single or infrequent consultation from out-of-state physician with licensed physician. Full license required of any physician providing services via technology.
Arkansas	Yes		
California MD/DO	Yes		No license required for consultations with a primary care physician licensed in California.
Colorado	Yes		Licensed Colorado physician may consult with physicians licensed in another state. Full license required to use telemedicine to diagnose and treat diseases.
Connecticut	Yes		In the case of electronic transmissions of radiographic images, license required for an out-of-state physician who provides, through an ongoing, regular, or contractual arrangement, official written reports of diagnostic evaluations of such images to Connecticut physicians or patients. No license required of a physician residing out of state who consults on an irregular basis with a licensed Connecticut physician, is located in-state, or is with a state medical school for educational or medical training purposes.
Delaware			No license required, if physician is licensed in another state and performs a consultation no more than six times a year.
DC		Yes	
Florida MD and DO	Yes		Physician licensed in another state, territory, or foreign country is permitted to examine the patient, take a history and physical, review laboratory tests and radiographs, and make recommendations about diagnosis and treatment to a licensed Florida physician. The term "consultation" does not include such physician's performance of any medical procedure on or the rendering of treatment to the patient. Full licensure required for out-of-state physicians using telemedicine to treat Florida residents.
Georgia	Yes		License required for out-of-state telemedicine.
Guam	Yes		Must hold license in state where physician resides.
Hawaii	Yes		Out-of-state consultant must be licensed in the state in which he/she resides; may not open an office (or appoint a place to meet patients or receive calls) in Hawaii.
Idaho			No license required for out-of-state physicians consulted by licensed Idaho physicians.
Illinois	Yes		Full license required.
Indiana	Yes		Will be updated soon.
Iowa			No license required for incidental consultation with out-of-state physicians by licensed Iowa physicians; out-of-state physician must be licensed if providing medical services to Iowa patients.
Kansas	Yes		License required if orders for services are issued for individuals located in Kansas. No license required for consultant licensed in another state who does not open an office or maintain a place to meet patients or receive calls in Kansas. No license required for services performed under supervision or by order of or referral from a licensed Kansas physician.
Kentucky	Yes		No license required for single or infrequent consultation from out-of-state physician with licensed physician. Full license required of any physician providing services via technology.
Louisiana	Yes		
Maine	Yes		No license required for incidental consultation with out-of-state physicians by licensed Maine physicians; out-of-state physician must be licensed if providing medical services to patients in Maine.
Maryland		Yes	Maryland license required, unless in consultation with a licensed Maryland physician on one specific patient.
Massachusetts			Full license required.
Michigan MD and DO		Yes	No license required for a physician living in and authorized to practice in another state or country who, in exceptional circumstances, is called for consultation or treatment by a Michigan health professional.
Minnesota	Yes		Telemedicine registration not required for physicians providing services in response to an emergency condition, services on an irregular or infrequent basis, or services as a consultant with a Minnesota-licensed physician who has ultimate authority over diagnosis and care of patient.
Mississippi	Yes		No license required for out-of-state physicians called for consultation by a licensed physician residing in Mississippi. Consultation period cannot exceed 5 days. Refer to introductory text to this table for more.

(continued on next page)

Table 21 (continued)
Regulations on the Practice of Telemedicine and Out-of-state Consulting Physicians

	Practice of Telemedicine		
	Has Adopted Regulations	Has Begun to Develop Regulations	Specific Licensure Restrictions on and/or Requirements for Out-of-state Consulting Physicians
Missouri	Yes		Licensed Missouri physician may consult with physicians licensed in another state. Full license required to use telemedicine to diagnose and treat diseases.
Montana	Yes		License required if an out-of-state consultant establishes a regular, direct physician/patient relationship.
Nebraska			Refer to Neb Rev Stat 38-2024 and 38-2025.
Nevada	Yes		Special purpose license required. Active license in home jurisdiction required.
Nevada DO	Yes		Licensure application required.
New Hampshire			License required if consultation is not made directly with a licensed New Hampshire physician or if consulting is more than incidental.
New Jersey		Yes	
New Mexico	Yes		Telemedicine license is required, with some exceptions; contact the Board for more information.
New York			New York license required.
North Carolina	Yes		North Carolina license required by state law.
North Dakota			North Dakota license required.
Ohio	Yes		Telemedicine license is required, with some exceptions; contact the Board for more information.
Oklahoma	Yes		License required for regular, ongoing treatment; license not required for occasional consultation.
Oregon	Yes		Full license required for telemedicine, teleradiology, or telemonitoring.
Pennsylvania		Yes	Pennsylvania license required.
Puerto Rico			
Rhode Island		Yes	Requirements exist for out-of-state consultants.
South Carolina			Must have permanent South Carolina license.
South Dakota	Yes		Any nonresident MD or DO who, while located outside South Dakota, provides diagnostic or treatment services through electronic means to a patient in this state under a contract with a health care provider, a clinic in this state that provides health services, or health care facility is engaged in the practice of medicine or osteopathy in South Dakota. Out-of-state MDs or DOs who consult on an irregular basis with a licensed South Dakota physician are not considered to practice in South Dakota.
Tennessee	Yes		Telemedicine license required of out-of-state physicians diagnosing or treating patients in Tennessee. Some exceptions granted.
Texas	Yes		Telemedicine license required for practice of medicine across state lines; visiting physician temporary license required for out-of-state physicians.
Utah	Yes		No license required of out-of-state physicians consulting with licensed Utah physician; full license required if consulting directly with patient by any means.
Vermont			Full license required.
Virgin Islands			
Virginia			Virginia license required if practice of medicine occurs in state.
Washington			May not set up an office, appoint a place for meeting patients, or receive calls within this state.
West Virginia	Yes		License required (with exceptions).
West Virginia DO			West Virginia license required.
Wisconsin	No		Wisconsin license required.
Wyoming	Yes		No license required of physicians residing in and licensed to practice medicine in another state or country called for consultation via telephone, electronic, or any other means by a licensed Wyoming physician. License required if consultations exceed one 7-day period in any 52-week period.

Note: *All information should be verified with the licensing board; medical licenses are granted to those physicians meeting all state requirements—at the discretion of the board.*

Regulations Related to Violations of Ethical Standards

The following table summarizes responses from state boards as to whether whether the board's statutes, rules or policies specifically refer to the AMA *Code of Medical Ethics* for violations of ethical standards (Table 22).

Opinion 1.01 of the Code, "Terminology" notes that "the term 'ethical' is used in opinions of the Council on Ethical and Judicial Affairs to refer to matters involving (1) moral principles or practices and (2) matters of social policy involving issues of morality in the practice of medicine. The term 'unethical' is used to refer to professional conduct which fails to conform to these moral standards or policies.

"Many of the Council's opinions lay out specific duties and obligations for physicians. Violation of these principles and opinions represents unethical conduct and may justify disciplinary action such as censure, suspension, or expulsion from medical society membership."

For more information on the AMA *Code of Medical Ethics*, see *www.ama-assn.org/go/ethics*.

Table 22
Regulations Related to Violations of Ethical Standards

	Reference to AMA Code of Ethics		
	Yes/No	Citation	Specific Language and/or Ccomments
Alabama			
Alaska	Yes	12 AAC 40.955.(a) ETHICAL STANDARDS	The Principles of Medical Ethics of the AMA on page xiv of the 2002-2003 Edition of the Council on Ethical and Judicial Affairs, *Code of Medical Ethics*, published by the AMA, are adopted by reference as the ethical standards for physicians and applies to all physicians subject to this chapter.
Arizona	No		
Arkansas			
California			
Colorado			
Connecticut	No		
Delaware			
DC	No		
Florida			
Georgia	No		
Guam			
Hawaii	Yes		
Idaho			
Illinois			
Indiana			
Iowa			
Kansas			
Kentucky	Yes	KRS 311.595(9), and 311.597(4)	
Louisiana			
Maine			
Maryland			
Massachusetts			
Michigan	No		An expert may rely on the AMA Code to explain the underpinnings of what he/she deems to be the controlling standard
Minnesota			
Mississippi			
Missouri			
Montana			
Nebraska			
Nevada			
New Hampshire	Yes		In the Board's rules
New Jersey		Yes	
New Mexico	Yes		"Determination of Medical Ethics" A. The board adopts the ethical standards set forth in the latest published version of the *Code of Medical Ethics*, current opinions with annotations of the Council on Ethical and Judicial Affairs of the AMA or its successor publication.
New York			

(continued on next page)

Table 22 (continued)
Regulations Related to Violations of Ethical Standards

	Reference to AMA Code of Ethics		Specific Language and/or Ccomments
	Yes/No	Citation	
North Carolina			
North Dakota			
Ohio			
Oklahoma			
Oregon	No	ORS 677.188 (4)(a)	"Unprofessional conduct" includes conduct or practice "contrary to recognized standards of ethics of the medical or podiatric profession" . . . The Board uses the AMA Code to interpret "recognized standards."
Pennsylvania	No		
Puerto Rico			
Rhode Island			
South Carolina	No	SECTION 40-47-70. Code of ethics. 40-47-110(13) Reg. 81-10(b) Reg. 81-60. Principles of Medical Ethics.	"A practitioner shall conduct himself or herself in accordance with the applicable codes of ethics adopted by the board in regulation"; "violated the code of medical ethics adopted by the board or has been found by the board to lack the ethical or professional competence to practice"; "violation of any of the principles of medical ethics as adopted by the Board."
South Dakota	.		
Tennessee	Yes		The Board adopted the AMA ethic in their rules.
Texas	No		
Utah			
Vermont	No		The Board routinely uses the AMA Code.
Virgin Islands			
Virginia			
Washington			
West Virginia	Yes	11 CSR 1A at 12.2(d).	
Wisconsin			
Wyoming	No		Considers the AMA Code when establishing the standard.

**Note: *All information should be verified with licensing board;
medical licenses are granted to those physicians meeting all
state requirements—at the discretion of the board.***

Section II.

Statistics of State Medical/Osteopathic Licensing Boards

Data in this section were taken from the AMA Physician Masterfile, an electronic database that tracks physicians' entire educational and professional careers, from medical school and graduate medical education (GME) through practice. Data include *only* full and unrestricted licenses; limited educational permits or licenses for resident physicians in GME programs are *not* included. Licenses issued to doctors of osteopathy (DOs) are also included.

Please note the following definitions:

Initial License—When a physician without *any* previous licensure receives the first license of his/her professional career.

New License—When a physician without previous licensure from a particular state receives a license from that state.

These two figures overlap, as all initial licenses are a subset of new licenses.

In 2008, 61,738 licenses were issued to doctors of medicine (MDs) and doctors of osteopathy (DOs) by medical licensing boards (see Table 23). Of these, 24,460 or 39.6%, were identified as initial licenses.

Table 24 shows a breakdown of total licenses awarded in 2008 by licensing jurisdiction, by US medical graduates and international medical graduates (IMGs).

Tables 25 through 27 present data on initial licensure. As previously noted, an initial license is the physician's first ever full and unrestricted license.

Table 25 shows the percentage of initial licenses awarded in a given jurisdiction. As previously noted, the national average for 2008 was 39.6%. In the states with higher percentages, then, the physician population is growing more rapidly than the national average.

Table 25 also breaks out the total initial licenses in each state by US medical school graduates and IMGs. Of the 24,460 physicians who received their initial licenses in 2008, 7,002 (28.6%) were issued to IMGs.

Table 26 provides an historical picture of the numbers of initial licenses awarded since 1950 and how the percentages have varied between US medical graduates and IMGs.

Table 23
Licenses Issued to Physicians by State Medical/Osteopathic Boards, 1975–2008

Year	Total New Licenses	Total Initial Licenses
1975	36,621	16,859
1976	38,488	17,724
1977	39,919	18,175
1978	41,457	19,393
1979	42,015	19,896
1980	41,112	18,172
1981	43,092	18,831
1982	43,543	17,605
1983	44,548	20,601
1984	43,681	18,340
1985	41,943	18,288
1986	43,375	19,528
1987	44,998	20,324
1988	44,969	21,235
1989	45,648	20,115
1990	44,341	20,853
1991	45,249	20,962
1992	45,132	19,760
1993	48,834	20,182
1994	49,912	20,857
1995	51,332	22,250
1996	55,716	23,920
1997	55,886	24,151
1998	56,237	23,419
1999	54,586	22,999
2000	51,866	19,581
2001	52,305	21,078
2002	52,877	20,383
2003	52,281	20,632
2004	55,435	22,599
2005	57,184	23,180
2006	61,724	24,287
2007	60,336	23,837
2008	61,738	24,460

In 1950, for example, only 5% of initial licensees were IMGs; in 2008, 29% were IMGs. The highest percentage of IMGs as initial licensees occurred in 1972 and 1973, with 46% and 44%, respectively (by 1979, however, the percentage had dropped back to 18%).

Table 27 provides an historical picture of the numbers of IMGs receiving initial licenses by state since 1975.

Table 24
Full Unrestricted Licenses (Whether Physician's Initial or Subsequent) Issued to MDs and DOs by State Medical/Osteopathic Boards, 2008

	Total	US Medical Graduates	IMGs	Percentage of Licenses Awarded to IMGs
Alabama	728	591	137	19
Alaska	252	222	30	12
Arizona	1,561	1,126	435	28
Arkansas	415	303	112	27
California	4,996	3,750	1,246	25
Colorado	1,017	898	119	12
Connecticut	1,011	608	403	40
Delaware	364	270	94	26
DC	632	473	159	25
Florida	2,921	1,850	1,071	37
Georgia	1,608	1,213	395	25
Hawaii	490	400	90	18
Idaho	464	406	58	13
Illinois	1,495	1,132	363	24
Indiana	1,604	1,133	471	29
Iowa	666	474	192	29
Kansas	662	502	160	24
Kentucky	969	736	233	24
Louisiana	725	513	212	29
Maine	439	337	102	23
Maryland	1,509	1,100	409	27
Massachusetts	2,312	1,694	618	27
Michigan	1,859	1,219	640	34
Minnesota	1,151	881	270	23
Mississippi	435	358	77	18
Missouri	1,341	1,015	326	24
Montana	272	243	29	11
Nebraska	563	489	74	13
Nevada	542	415	127	23
New Hampshire	483	352	131	27
New Jersey	1,681	1,054	627	37
New Mexico	569	440	129	23
New York	4,297	2,902	1,395	32
North Carolina	1,981	1,567	414	21
North Dakota	233	174	59	25
Ohio	2,127	1,523	604	28
Oklahoma	751	550	201	27
Oregon	786	655	131	17
Pennsylvania	2,891	1,974	917	32
Puerto Rico	235	138	97	41
Rhode Island	178	126	52	29
South Carolina	836	649	187	22
South Dakota	270	216	54	20
Tennessee	1,247	1,012	235	19
Texas	3,521	2,516	1,005	29
Utah	699	601	98	14
Vermont	222	198	24	11
Virginia	2,033	1,489	544	27
Virgin Islands	5	5	0	0
Washington	1,670	1,344	326	20
West Virginia	466	316	150	32
Wisconsin	1,324	960	364	27
Wyoming	230	192	38	17
Total	**61,738**	**45,082**	**16,434**	**27 (avg)**

Table 25
Initial Licenses Issued to MDs and DOs by State Medical/Osteopathic Boards, 2008

	Total	US Medical Graduates	IMGs	Initial Licenses Awarded as Percentage of Full Unrestricted Licenses (Table 24)
Alabama	304	253	51	42
Alaska	19	16	3	8
Arizona	363	253	110	23
Arkansas	138	84	54	33
California	2,771	2,148	623	55
Colorado	279	244	35	27
Connecticut	395	173	222	39
Delaware	75	55	20	21
DC	194	151	43	31
Florida	818	435	383	28
Georgia	476	354	122	30
Hawaii	120	93	27	24
Idaho	36	33	3	8
Illinois	774	577	197	52
Indiana	643	427	216	40
Iowa	228	142	86	34
Kansas	178	128	50	27
Kentucky	229	155	74	24
Louisiana	343	248	95	47
Maine	80	54	26	18
Maryland	495	335	160	33
Massachusetts	1,223	899	324	53
Michigan	1,001	563	438	54
Minnesota	579	442	137	50
Mississippi	121	95	26	28
Missouri	517	397	120	39
Montana	19	17	2	7
Nebraska	251	234	17	45
Nevada	57	28	29	11
New Hampshire	103	56	47	21
New Jersey	515	248	267	31
New Mexico	141	94	47	25
New York	2,633	1,849	784	61
North Carolina	607	504	103	31
North Dakota	28	17	11	12
Ohio	1,080	774	306	51
Oklahoma	272	167	105	36
Oregon	205	164	41	26
Pennsylvania	1,475	992	483	51
Puerto Rico	184	97	87	78
Rhode Island	28	17	11	16
South Carolina	242	196	46	29
South Dakota	20	13	7	7
Tennessee	395	321	74	32
Texas	1,423	1,177	246	40
Utah	297	262	35	42
Vermont	52	47	5	23
Virginia	836	627	209	42
Virgin Islands	5	5	0	100
Washington	448	334	114	27
West Virginia	128	78	50	27
Wisconsin	597	412	185	45
Wyoming	27	12	15	12
Total	**24,460**	**17,458**	**7,002**	**39.6 (avg)**

Table 26
Initial Licenses Issued to MDs and DOs by State Medical/Osteopathic Boards, 1950-2008

Year	Total	US Medical Graduates		IMGs	
1950	6,002	5,694	95%	308	5%
1951	6,273	5,923	94%	350	6%
1952	6,885	6,316	92%	569	8%
1953	7,276	6,591	91%	685	9%
1954	7,917	7,145	90%	772	10%
1955	7,737	6,830	88%	907	12%
1956	7,463	6,611	89%	852	11%
1957	7,455	6,441	86%	1,014	14%
1958	7,809	6,643	85%	1,166	15%
1959	8,269	6,643	80%	1,626	20%
1960	8,030	6,611	82%	1,419	18%
1961	8,023	6,443	80%	1,580	20%
1962	8,005	6,648	83%	1,357	17%
1963	8,283	6,832	82%	1,451	18%
1964	7,911	6,605	83%	1,306	17%
1965	9,147	7,619	83%	1,528	17%
1966	8,851	7,217	82%	1,634	18%
1967	9,424	7,343	78%	2,081	22%
1968	9,766	7,581	78%	2,185	22%
1969	9,978	7,671	77%	2,307	23%
1970	11,032	8,016	73%	3,016	27%
1971	12,257	7,943	65%	4,314	35%
1972	14,476	7,815	54%	6,661	46%
1973	16,689	9,270	56%	7,419	44%
1974	16,706	10,093	60%	6,613	40%
1975	16,859	10,794	64%	6,065	36%
1976	17,724	11,288	64%	6,436	36%
1977	18,175	12,324	68%	5,851	32%
1978	19,393	14,815	76%	4,578	24%
1979	19,896	16,330	82%	3,566	18%
1980	18,172	14,862	82%	3,310	18%
1981	18,831	15,700	83%	3,131	17%
1982	17,605	13,409	76%	4,196	24%
1983	20,601	15,848	77%	4,753	23%
1984	18,340	14,246	78%	4,094	22%
1985	18,288	15,239	83%	3,049	17%
1986	19,528	16,592	85%	2,936	15%
1987	20,324	17,096	84%	3,228	16%
1988	21,235	18,005	85%	3,230	15%
1989	20,115	17,366	86%	2,749	14%
1990	20,853	17,254	83%	3,599	17%
1991	20,962	16,959	81%	4,003	19%
1992	19,760	16,008	81%	3,752	19%
1993	20,182	15,805	78%	4,377	22%
1994	20,857	15,961	77%	4,896	23%
1995	22,520	17,201	76%	5,319	24%
1996	23,920	17,486	73%	6,434	27%
1997	24,151	16,714	69%	7,069	31%
1998	23,419	17,786	76%	5,633	24%
1999	22,999	17,700	77%	5,299	23%
2000	19,581	14,586	74%	4,995	26%
2001	21,078	15,392	73%	5,686	27%
2002	20,383	14,888	73%	5,495	27%
2003	20,632	15,019	73%	5,613	27%
2004	22,599	16,239	72%	6,360	28%
2005	23,180	16,391	71%	6,789	29%
2006	24,287	17,506	72%	6,781	28%
2007	23,837	17,018	71%	6,819	29%
2008	24,460	17,458	71%	7,002	29%

Table 27
Initial Licenses Issued to International Medical Graduates by State Medical/Osteopathic Boards, 1975-2008

	1975	1980	1985	1990	1995	2000	2005	2007	2008
Alabama	1	0	8	11	136	28	73	58	51
Alaska	1	0	0	1	15	1	3	3	3
Arizona	20	16	17	14	8	28	80	108	110
Arkansas	8	5	9	13	31	27	48	51	54
California	212	276	243	355	435	392	701	730	623
Colorado	6	6	18	29	6	15	22	23	35
Connecticut	13	54	71	23	11	146	169	213	222
Delaware	9	3	4	9	4	16	25	17	20
DC	426	59	45	19	13	49	44	41	43
Florida	325	114	114	156	155	204	333	433	383
Georgia	74	165	113	38	67	62	106	96	122
Hawaii	14	9	6	15	14	9	26	18	27
Idaho	0	1	0	0	0	1	2	0	3
Illinois	481	94	75	369	631	360	393	424	197
Indiana	46	58	85	50	2	412	228	218	216
Iowa	71	36	132	49	107	73	71	65	86
Kansas	25	23	12	31	122	25	53	30	50
Kentucky	30	30	2	20	38	53	69	76	74
Louisiana	11	21	26	3	35	70	97	74	95
Maine	197	172	3	14	21	11	27	33	26
Maryland	258	244	125	239	213	0	127	152	160
Massachusetts	199	170	42	151	202	208	247	284	324
Michigan	565	146	195	31	431	323	474	457	438
Minnesota	39	16	49	38	50	84	80	135	137
Mississippi	9	5	0	5	0	15	32	24	26
Missouri	124	30	20	16	63	61	77	90	120
Montana	0	4	1	0	3	0	2	2	2
Nebraska	20	30	22	35	5	16	16	23	17
Nevada	5	4	0	1	5	17	34	36	29
New Hampshire	22	4	5	4	38	6	25	41	47
New Jersey	139	262	324	318	321	199	262	234	267
New Mexico	14	11	11	26	7	27	55	47	47
New York	805	594	352	975	640	683	724	767	784
North Carolina	66	19	35	18	57	56	90	102	103
North Dakota	45	20	6	0	6	8	9	8	11
Ohio	183	70	71	43	63	444	309	294	306
Oklahoma	30	72	39	20	25	42	73	86	105
Oregon	14	13	3	6	10	39	24	35	41
Pennsylvania	490	137	253	107	390	342	399	444	483
Puerto Rico	157	4	46	25	97	—	301	—	87
Rhode Island	7	11	20	11	17	30	29	12	11
South Carolina	2	13	1	2	160	20	25	24	46
South Dakota	3	12	5	0	6	3	7	11	7
Tennessee	18	23	20	25	57	48	66	64	74
Texas	201	100	49	54	18	54	190	183	246
Utah	4	1	12	36	237	16	26	26	35
Vermont	46	0	1	3	3	5	6	2	5
Virginia	327	49	43	49	79	113	235	209	240
Washington	22	23	263	30	89	53	83	122	114
West Virginia	119	38	14	35	23	13	35	36	50
Wisconsin	18	33	33	75	136	86	150	145	185
Wyoming	5	10	6	2	1	2	7	13	15
Total	**5,926**	**3,310**	**3,049**	**3,599**	**5,303**	**4,995**	**6,789**	**6,819**	**7,002**

Section III.

Medical Licensing Examinations and Organizations

The United States
Medical Licensing Examination® (USMLE®)

National Board of Medical Examiners
Philadelphia, Pennsylvania

The United States Medical Licensing Examination®
(USMLE®) is a three-step examination for medical licensure in the United States. It is designed to assess a physician's ability to apply knowledge, concepts, and principles,
and to demonstrate fundamental patient-centered skills,
that are important in health and disease and that constitute
the basis of safe and effective patient care. The USMLE is
a single examination with three Steps. Each Step is complementary to the others; no Step can stand alone in the
assessment of readiness for medical licensure. The
USMLE is sponsored by the Federation of State Medical
Boards (FSMB) and the National Board of Medical
Examiners® (NBME®).

A Composite Committee, appointed by the FSMB and
NBME, governs the USMLE. The Composite Committee
establishes rules for the USMLE program. Membership
includes representatives from the FSMB, NBME, the
Educational Commission for Foreign Medical Graduates
(ECFMG®), and the American public.

In the United States and its territories, the individual medical licensing authorities ("state medical boards") of the
various jurisdictions grant a license to practice medicine.
Each medical licensing authority sets its own rules and
regulations and requires passing an examination that
demonstrates qualification for licensure. Results of the
USMLE are reported to these authorities for use in
granting the initial license to practice medicine. The
USMLE provides them with a common evaluation system
for applicants for medical licensure. Because individual
medical licensing authorities make their own decisions
regarding use of USMLE results, licensure applicants
should obtain complete information from the licensing
authority. Also, the FSMB can provide general information
on medical licensure.

Note: Portions of this chapter reprinted with permission from the
USMLE 2009 Bulletin of Information, copyright © 2008 by the
Federation of State Medical Boards of the United States, Inc, and the
National Board of Medical Examiners®; and also from the *2007
NBME Annual Report*, copyright © 2008 by the National Board of
Medical Examiners®.

The Three Steps of the USMLE:
Step 1, Step 2, and Step 3

Step 1 assesses whether medical school students or graduates can understand and apply important concepts of the
sciences basic to the practice of medicine, with special
emphasis on principles and mechanisms underlying health,
disease, and modes of therapy. Step 1 ensures mastery of
not only the sciences that provide a foundation for the safe
and competent practice of medicine in the present, but also
the scientific principles required for maintenance of competence through lifelong learning.

Step 2 has two separately administered components, the
Clinical Knowledge component (Step 2 CK) and the
Clinical Skills component (Step 2 CS). The Clinical Skills
component became a part of Step 2 in June 2004. Step 2
assesses whether medical school students or graduates can
understand and apply the knowledge, skills, and understanding of clinical science considered essential for the
provision of patient care under supervision and includes
emphasis on health promotion and disease prevention. The
inclusion of Step 2 in the USMLE sequence is intended to
ensure that due attention is devoted to principles of clinical
sciences and basic patient-centered skills that provide the
foundation for safe and competent medical practice.

Step 3 assesses whether physicians can apply the medical
knowledge and understanding of biomedical and clinical
science considered essential for the unsupervised practice
of medicine, with emphasis on patient management in
ambulatory settings. The inclusion of Step 3 in the
USMLE sequence ensures that attention is devoted to the
importance of assessing the knowledge of physicians who
are assuming independent responsibility for delivering
general medical care to patients.

USMLE Eligibility Requirements
and Examination Policies

To be eligible to sit for USMLE Step 1, Step 2 CK, and
Step 2 CS, an applicant must be in one of the following
categories at the time of application and on the examination day:

- A medical student officially enrolled in, or a graduate of, a US or Canadian medical school program leading to the MD degree that is accredited by the Liaison Committee on Medical Education (LCME)

- A medical student officially enrolled in, or a graduate of, a US medical school program leading to the DO degree that is accredited by the American Osteopathic Association (AOA)

- A medical student officially enrolled in, or a graduate of, a medical school outside the United States and Canada and eligible for examination by the ECFMG for its certificate

To be eligible to sit for USMLE Step 3, an applicant must meet all of the following requirements:

- Obtain the MD degree (or its equivalent) or the DO degree

- Obtain a passing performance on Steps 1 and 2 (for those required to take Step 2 CS, both the CS and the CK components of Step 2 must be passed in order to be eligible to register for Step 3; see the current USMLE *Bulletin of Information* at *www.usmle.org* for a detailed description of who is required to take and pass Step 2 CS to be eligible to register for Step 3)

- If a graduate of a medical school outside the United States and Canada, obtain certification by the ECFMG or successfully complete a Fifth Pathway program (see page 28 for more information)

- Meet the requirements for taking Step 3 set by the medical licensing authority to which the applicant is applying

The USMLE program recommends that, for Step 3 eligibility, licensing authorities require the completion, or near completion, of at least 1 training year in a GME program accredited by the Accreditation Council for Graduate Medical Education (ACGME) or the AOA. Applicants should contact the FSMB or the individual licensing authority for complete information on Step 3 eligibility requirements in the state where they plan to be licensed.

Medical students or graduates planning to take USMLE must obtain the most recent information from the appropriate registration entity (see page 94) before applying for the examination. See the USMLE Web site at *www.usmle.org* for updated information.

Computer-based Testing

Through computer-based testing (CBT), continuous test administration of the USMLE Step 1, Step 2 CK, and Step 3 is available to all examinees. Prometric® provides scheduling and test centers for the USMLE. The Step 1 and Step 2 CK examinations are administered worldwide; the Step 3 examination is administered only in the United States.

Step 2 CS Testing

USMLE Step 2 CS is administered at five regional Clinical Skills Evaluation Centers in the United States:

- Atlanta, Georgia
- Chicago, Illinois
- Houston, Texas
- Philadelphia, Pennsylvania
- Los Angeles, California

Step 2 CS is offered regularly throughout the year at these five sites.

Description of the Examinations

Step 1, Step 2 CK, and Step 3 are administered in sessions of 8 or 9 hours, broken up into sections, or "blocks." The computer keeps track of overall session time, including break time and time allocated for each block of the test. Step 2 CS consists of 12 patient cases. Examinees have 15 minutes for each patient encounter and 10 minutes to record the patient note. The testing session is approximately 8 hours. Further information on examination content and sample test materials for all three steps of the USMLE are available at the USMLE Web site (*www.usmle.org*).

Step 1

Step 1 has 336 multiple-choice test items, divided into seven 60-minute blocks, administered in one 8-hour testing session. It includes test questions in anatomy, behavioral sciences, biochemistry, microbiology, pathology, pharmacology, and physiology, as well as interdisciplinary topics such as nutrition, genetics, and aging. Step 1 is a broadly based, integrated examination. Test questions commonly require examinees to interpret graphic and tabular material, to identify gross and microscopic pathologic and normal specimens, and to apply basic science knowledge to clinical problems. Step 1 is constructed according to an integrated content outline that organizes basic science material along two dimensions: system and process.

Step 2 CK

Step 2 CK has approximately 370 multiple-choice test items, divided into eight 60-minute blocks, administered in one 9-hour testing session. It includes test questions in internal medicine, obstetrics and gynecology, pediatrics, preventive medicine, psychiatry, surgery, and other areas relevant to provision of care under supervision. The majority of the test questions describe clinical situations and require that examinees provide a diagnosis, prognosis, indication of underlying mechanisms of disease, or the next step in medical care, including preventive measures. Step 2 CK is a broadly based, integrated examination. Interpretation of tables and laboratory data, imaging studies, photographs of gross and microscopic pathologic specimens, and results of other diagnostic studies is frequently required. Step 2 CK is constructed according to an integrated content outline that organizes clinical science material along two dimensions: physician task and disease category.

Step 2 CS

Step 2 CS uses standardized patients, ie, people trained to portray real patients. Examinees are expected to establish rapport with the standardized patients, elicit pertinent historical information from them, perform focused physical examinations, answer questions, and provide counseling when appropriate. After each interaction with a standardized patient, examinees record pertinent history and physical examination findings, list diagnostic impressions, and outline plans for further evaluation, if necessary. The cases cover common and important situations that a physician is likely to encounter in clinics, doctors' offices, emergency departments, and hospital settings in the United States. The sample of cases selected for each examination reflects a balance of cases that is fair and equitable across all examinations. On any examination day, the set of cases will differ from the combination presented the day before or the following day, but each set of cases has a comparable degree of difficulty. The criteria used to create individual examinations focus primarily on presenting complaints and conditions. Presentation categories include, but are not

limited to, cardiovascular, constitutional, gastrointestinal, genitourinary, musculoskeletal, neurological, psychiatric, respiratory, and women's health.

Three subcomponents of Step 2 CS are assessed: (1) Integrated Clinical Encounter, which includes data-gathering skills, including history taking and physical examination, and a patient note; (2) Communication and Interpersonal Skills; and (3) Spoken English Proficiency. Examinees are assessed on their data gathering, physical examination, and communication skills (including spoken English) by the standardized patient, and on their ability to complete the patient note by physician raters.

Examinees must pass all three components in a single administration to obtain the overall designation of passing Step 2 CS. Step 2 CS results are reported as pass or fail, with no numerical scores.

Step 3

Step 3 has approximately 480 multiple-choice test items, divided into blocks of 35 to 50 items, with 45 to 60 minutes to complete each block. In addition, Step 3 has nine computer-based case simulations, with approximately 25 minutes to complete each case. Step 3 is administered in two 8-hour testing sessions.

Step 3 is organized along two principal dimensions: clinical encounter frame and physician task. Step 3 content reflects a data-based model of generalist medical practice in the United States. Encounter frames capture the essential features of circumstances surrounding physicians' clinical activity with patients. They range from encounters with patients seen for the first time for nonemergency problems, to encounters with regular patients seen in the context of continued care, to patient encounters in (life-threatening) emergency situations. Encounters occur in clinics, offices, skilled nursing care facilities, hospitals and emergency departments, and on the telephone.

Step 3 includes Primum® computer-based case simulations (CCS), a test format developed by the NBME that allows the physician taking the test to provide care for a simulated patient. The test-taker decides which diagnostic information to obtain and how to treat and monitor the patient's progress. The computer records each step taken in caring for the patient and scores overall performance. This format permits assessment of clinical decision-making skills in a more realistic and integrated manner than multiple-choice formats.

In the CCS cases, the test-taker may request information from the history and physical examination; order laboratory studies, procedures, and consultants; and start medications and other therapies. Any of the thousands of possible entries that are typed on the "order sheet" are processed and verified by the "clerk." When the test-taker has confirmed that there is nothing further to do, he or she decides when to reevaluate the patient by advancing simulated time. As time passes, the patient's condition changes based on the underlying problem and interventions taken; results of tests are reported and results of interventions must be monitored. The test-taker can suspend the movement of simulated time to consider next steps. While one cannot go back in time, orders can be changed to reflect an updated management plan.

The patient's chart contains, in addition to the order sheet, the reports resulting from orders. By selecting the appropriate chart tabs, the test-taker can review vital signs, progress notes, nurses' notes, and test results. He or she may care for and move the patient among the office, home, emergency department, intensive care unit, and hospital ward.

Preparation for the Examinations

There are no test preparation courses affiliated with or sanctioned by the USMLE program. Information on such courses is not available from the ECFMG, FSMB, NBME, USMLE Secretariat, or medical licensing authorities.

USMLE Steps are broad in scope and are designed to measure the prospective physician's ability to apply knowledge. The best preparation for the USMLE is a general, thorough review of the content reflected in the descriptions for each Step (available at the USMLE Web site).

USMLE Minimum Passing Scores

The USMLE program recommends a minimum passing score for each Step of the USMLE. Minimum passing scores are based on achievement of specified levels of proficiency established prior to administration of examinations. Statistical procedures are employed to ensure that for each Step, the level of proficiency required to pass remains uniform across forms of the examination. As noted in the

USMLE *Bulletin of Information* at *www.usmle.org*, the score required to meet the recommended level of proficiency is reviewed periodically and may be adjusted without prior notice. Notice of adjustments is posted at the USMLE Web site.

In reviewing standards for USMLE examinations, the USMLE Step Committees employ information gathered from a number of sources, including standard-setting surveys. These surveys, which seek opinions on the appropriateness of current USMLE pass/fail standards for each of the Steps, are sent to random samples of examinees, directors of basic and clinical science courses and clinical clerkships, associate deans for academic and student affairs, directors and chief residents from residency programs, members of USMLE test material development committees, executive directors and presidents of all state medical boards, and members of the NBME Board and FSMB Board of Directors.

In addition to surveys, USMLE Step Committees consider the results of content review by standard setting panels. These panels typically consist of physicians who are not otherwise involved in the USMLE program. These panels review the content of the Step examinations and, through a series of exercises, provide data that reflect their opinions on minimally acceptable levels of performance.

Step 1

The USMLE Web site provides details on the performance of examinees taking Step 1 in 2007 and 2008. Data for 2008 are based upon examinees whose results were reported through February 4, 2009. Approximately 17,000 and 17,500 first-time takers from US and Canadian medical schools that grant the MD degree were tested in 2007 and 2008, respectively. First-time takers from non-US/Canadian medical schools numbered 15,762 and 14,889 for the same years. The pass rates for first-time takers from MD-granting US and Canadian medical schools were 95% in 2007 and 94% in 2008. Because failing examinees generally retake Step 1, the ultimate passing rate across test administrations is expected to increase to approximately 99% for this same group.

Step 2 CK

The USMLE Web site provides details on the performance of examinees taking Step 2 CK in the 2006-2007 and 2007-2008 academic years. First-time takers from US and Canadian medical schools granting the MD degree numbered approximately 16,500 for both 2006-2007 and

2007-2008. First-time takers from non-US/Canadian medical schools numbered 12,584 and 12,847, respectively. The pass rates for first-time takers from MD-granting US and Canadian medical schools were 96% for both academic years. As noted with Step 1, given the opportunity for this same group to repeat the examination, the ultimate Step 2 CK passing rate across test administrations is expected to increase to approximately 99% for this same group.

Step 2 CS

The USMLE Web site provides details on the performance of examinees taking Step 2 CS in the 2006-2007 and 2007-2008 academic years. First-time takers from US and Canadian medical schools granting the MD degree numbered 16,769 for 2006-2007 and 16,715 for 2007-2008, with passing rates of 97% for both years. First-time takers from non-US/Canadian medical schools numbered 14,439 and 13,787 during these two periods. The respective passing rates for this group were 77% and 72%.

Examinees taking Step 2 CS must pass three separate subcomponents in order to record an overall pass on Step 2 CS. The three subcomponents are: Integrated Clinical Encounter (ICE), Communication and Interpersonal Skills (CIS), and Spoken English Proficiency (SEP).

Step 3

The USMLE Web site provides details on the performance of examinees taking Step 3 in 2007 and 2008. Data for 2008 are based upon examinees whose results were reported through February 4, 2009. First-time takers who were graduates of MD-granting schools in the US and Canada numbered 16,633 in 2007 and 17,245 in 2008. First-time takers who were graduates of non-US/Canadian medical schools numbered 9,384 and 9,376, respectively, for the same years. The pass rate for first-time takers who were graduates of MD-granting US and Canadian medical schools was 96% in 2007 and 95% in 2008. As with Step 1 and Step 2 CK, the ultimate Step 3 passing rate, accounting for repeat attempts, is expected to increase to approximately 99% for this same group.

Step 3 Standard Setting

Performance standards for Step 3 were reviewed in 2008. Changes in the Step 3 minimum passing score are described on the USMLE Web site.

The Comprehensive Review of USMLE

In 2004, the USMLE Composite Committee called for the formation of a Planning Task Force to plan a review of USMLE purpose, design, format and timing. Over the next year the Planning Task Force developed a plan for gathering opinion on the value and usefulness of the current program, using surveys and a series of focus groups with a wide range of stakeholders. Throughout 2006, focus groups were held to gather feedback from members of the medical licensing community, medical student organizations, and members of the undergraduate and graduate medical education community. Surveys were also developed to assess key stakeholders' opinions as to the usefulness and quality of the current USMLE program. Surveys were sent to executives and presidents of state licensing authorities; medical school deans, academic affairs deans and student affairs deans; national and local representatives of medical student organizations; selected foreign medical school representatives; residency program directors; and samples of examinees.

The Planning Task Force also proposed the appointment of a committee charged with beginning the review of the program. This group, the Committee to Evaluate the USMLE Program (CEUP), began its work in late 2006. The committee issued its final report to the Composite Committee in spring 2008. The recommendations included in the report outline a series of steps to enhance the value and utility of the USMLE program, and are listed at the USMLE Web site.

The Composite Committee met to discuss the CEUP recommendations in May 2008. The Composite Committee broadly concurred with the CEUP's report, endorsing the first three of its recommendations in their entirety and directing staff to conduct the research necessary to fulfill the others. The executive summary of the CEUP report is available at the USMLE Web site.

The Composite Committee identified guiding principles for the USMLE going forward. In broad strokes, these principles state that the primary purpose of the USMLE is to inform the medical licensing process by assessing the competencies of physicians wishing to practice medicine within the United States. The competencies considered central to safe and effective patient care are dynamic; therefore the USMLE should be responsive as national consensus about core competencies evolves. Furthermore, the USMLE must provide reliable measures of an aspiring physician's competencies and allow reasonable and valid interpretations.

Secondary uses of USMLE data should not adversely affect the USMLE program. Finally, any redesign of the USMLE should remain sensitive to the costs to students and other examinees and to administrative challenges.

Communicating About USMLE

Complete information on USMLE is available at the USMLE Web site. Table 28 provides contact information specific to the various Steps. General inquiries regarding the USMLE or inquires for the USMLE Secretariat may be directed to the NBME or the USMLE Secretariat:

USMLE Secretariat
3750 Market St
Philadelphia, PA 19104-3190
(215) 590-9700
www.usmle.org

Table 28
Contact Information for USMLE

Examination	Type of Applicant	Registration Entity to Contact
Step 1 or Step 2 (CK or CS)	Students and graduates of medical school programs in the US and Canada accredited by the Liaison Committee on Medical Education or students and graduates of medical schools in the US and Canada accredited by the American Osteopathic Association	**NBME** Examinee Support Services, 3750 Market St Philadelphia, PA 19104-3190 (215) 590-9700 (215) 590-9457 Fax E-mail: *webmail@nbme.org* *www.nbme.org*
Step 1 or Step 2 (CK or CS)	Students and graduates of medical schools outside the US and Canada	**ECFMG** 3624 Market St Philadelphia, PA 19104-2685 (215) 386-5900 (215) 386-9196 Fax E-mail: *info@ecfmg.org* *www.ecfmg.org*
Step 3	All medical school graduates who have passed Step 1 and Step 2	**FSMB** Department of Examination Services PO Box 619850 Dallas, TX 75261-9850 (817) 868-4041 (817) 868-4098 Fax E-mail: *usmle@fsmb.org* *www.fsmb.org* – or – **Medical licensing authority**

The Federation of State Medical Boards (FSMB) of the United States, Inc

The Federation of State Medical Boards of the United States, Inc (FSMB) is a nonprofit organization composed of the 70 state medical boards of the US and its territories. The FSMB works closely with state medical boards to improve the quality, safety, and integrity of US health care by promoting high standards for physician licensure and practice.

The primary responsibility of each medical licensing board is to protect the public through the regulation of physicians and other health care providers. Within the United States, the organization and activities of each board are determined by state statute, usually referred to as a medical practice act. In general, each state medical board has the authority to license physicians, regulate the practice of medicine, and discipline those who violate the medical practice act.

Physician Data Center

The Federation Physician Data Center is a central repository for formal actions taken against physicians by state licensing and disciplinary boards, the Department of Defense, the US Department of Health and Human Services, and a growing number of international regulatory organizations. The Data Center offers two services used in performing credentialing functions or pre-employment background checks: the *Board Action Data Search* and the *Disciplinary Alert Service*. Both of these services are considered primary source-equivalent by National Committee for Quality Assurance and The Joint Commission. The Data Center contains more than 156,000 board actions related to approximately 46,000 physicians dating to the 1960s. This information is available to licensing and disciplinary boards, the military, governmental and private agencies, and organizations involved in the employment and/or credentialing of physicians. The public can access a national consolidated database of state medical board disciplinary data at *www.docinfo.org* for a nominal search fee.

Licensure and Assessment Services

In the United States and its territories, a license to practice medicine is a privilege granted only by the individual medical licensing authority of a state or jurisdiction. Each authority sets its own rules and regulations, and each requires successful completion of an examination or certification demonstrating qualification for licensure.

The FSMB, in collaboration with the National Board of Medical Examiners (see page 99), offers two service packages used by medical licensing authorities for making licensure decisions: The United States Medical Licensing Examination (USMLE™) and the Post-Licensure Assessment System (PLAS).

The USMLE is a 3-step examination taken by individuals preparing for initial medical licensure in the United States. With steps designed to be taken at different times during medical education and training, the USMLE provides a common pathway for evaluating an individual's ability to apply medical knowledge, concepts, and principles to patient care and to demonstrate fundamental patient-centered skills that are important in health and disease and that constitute the basis of safe and effective patient care. (See page 90 for more information on USMLE.)

The Post-Licensure Assessment System (PLAS), established in 1998, is a joint program of the FSMB and the National Board of Medical Examiners (NBME). The PLAS provides comprehensive services to medical licensing authorities for use in assessing the ongoing clinical competence of licensed physicians. (More information on PLAS is provided on page 98.)

Federation Credentials Verification Service (FCVS)

The Federation Credentials Verification Service (FCVS) was launched in 1996 to provide a centralized, uniform process for state medical boards to obtain a verified, primary-source record of physicians' and physician assistants' medical credentials. This service is designed to lighten the workload of credentialing staff and reduce duplication of effort by gathering, verifying, and permanently storing the physician's credentials in a central repository at the FSMB's offices. FCVS obtains primary source verification of medical education, postgraduate training, examination history, board action history, board specialty certification, and identity. This repository of information allows a physician to establish a confidential, lifetime professional portfolio with FCVS which can be forwarded, at the physician's request, to any state medical board that has established an agreement with FCVS as well as other health care entities. To date, more than 100,000 physicians have used FCVS.

FCVS's Student Records program provides a central repository for medical training information, housing and verifying resident training records from closed training programs. This repository of information allows physicians to continue obtaining verification of training for state licensure and hospital and managed care privileging.

To request an FCVS application, receive more detailed information about the credentialing process, or request a roster of the state medical boards that accept FCVS documents, call toll-free (888) ASK-FCVS (888 275-3287), access the FSMB Web site at *www.fsmb.org*, or send an e-mail to *fcvs@fsmb.org*. For more information about FCVS's Student Records program, call (817) 868-5084, or e-mail *nlloyd@fsmb.org*.

Government Relations and Policy

The FSMB monitors federal and state legislation and regulatory policies that affect medical licensure and discipline. The FSMB Government Relations and Policy Department identifies current legislative trends and facilitates communication among member medical boards on issues of mutual interest. The department helps state medical boards develop legislative and administrative strategies to implement FSMB policy initiatives through model policy proposals, research assistance, written and oral testimony, and advocacy campaigns. The FSMB has played a key role in state and national debates on many prominent issues, including physician mobility and emergency preparedness, international medical education, sexual boundaries issues, Internet prescribing, physician profiling, pain management, oversight of resident physicians, complementary and alternative medicine, and the regulation of office-based surgery.

Publications

The FSMB leverages print and electronic publications to inform its membership, the health care community, and the public about medical licensing, regulation, discipline, and medical trends. Model guidelines and recommendations for handling key issues—such as Internet prescribing, pain management, and international medical education—are set forth in published policy documents available online or in print.

On a quarterly basis, the FSMB publishes the *Journal of Medical Licensure and Discipline*, which is distributed to FSMB membership, libraries, medical schools, and subscribers around the world. Member boards and their staffs are served by the bimonthly newsletter *Newsline* and the weekly e-mail publication *Boardnet News*.

The FSMB also publishes all of its policy documents, organizational updates, and the United States Medical Licensing Examination applications, all of which are available online at *www.fsmb.org*.

Education

The FSMB offers a variety of educational forums designed to assist state medical boards in carrying out their mission of public protection. The FSMB Annual Meeting is an intensive three-day program that brings together medical regulators from around the world to discuss trends impacting public safety. To meet the changing needs of its member boards, the FSMB offers Web-based educational programs that bring boards together with national experts to discuss current issues in medical regulation. Recent webinars have addressed issues in pain management and the prescribing of controlled substances, sexual boundary issues, and disruptive behavior by physicians. Other program offerings include workshops for medical board attorneys and a comprehensive overview of FSMB programs and services for executives new to medical boards. CME and CLE credits are available through various program offerings.

Post-Licensure Assessment System (PLAS)

The Post-Licensure Assessment System (PLAS) is a joint program of the FSMB and the National Board of Medical Examiners (NBME®). The PLAS provides a comprehensive inventory of assessment tools that are useful in evaluating the clinical competence of licensed or previously licensed physicians.

Assessing Medical Knowledge: The Special Purpose Examination (SPEX)

The Special Purpose Examination (SPEX) is an examination of current knowledge requisite for the general undifferentiated practice of medicine and is intended for physicians who hold or have held a valid, unrestricted license to practice medicine in a US or Canadian jurisdiction. Licensing boards may require SPEX for licensure by endorsement applicants who are some years beyond passage of an initial licensing examination or to evaluate the cognitive knowledge of physicians seeking licensure reinstatement or reactivation after some period of professional inactivity. Physicians who hold a current, unrestricted license to practice in a US or Canadian jurisdiction can take SPEX independent of any request or approval from a medical licensing board.

The SPEX focuses on a core of clinical knowledge and relevant underlying basic science principles deemed necessary to form a reasonable foundation for the safe and effective practice of medicine. The content is organized along two primary dimensions: clinical encounter categories and physician tasks. Scores are reported directly to the licensing boards for which SPEX is taken, if applicable, and to the examinee. At the request of an examinee, the FSMB will provide certified transcripts of SPEX scores to additional licensing boards.

For more information about the SPEX, call the FSMB Examination Hotline at (817) 868-4041 or consult the FSMB Web site at *www.fsmb.org*.

Multi-modal Clinical Competence Assessment Resources

The PLAS also provides diverse, state-of-the-art assessment modalities that, when administered together, generate comprehensive and pertinent data regarding a physician's medical knowledge, clinical judgment, and patient management skills in the current or intended area of practice.

Assessment resources currently available through PLAS include Primum® Computer-based Case Simulations; standardized, practice-relevant, multiple-choice exams; and multiple-choice topic module exams. These tools are utilized by physician evaluation and remediation programs around the country to complement local, performance-based methods of assessment, such as medical record reviews, peer (preceptor) assessment and feedback, patient evaluations, and case-based evaluations of physician care.

A comprehensive assessment will help determine the strengths and weaknesses a physician has in areas such as practice-relevant medical knowledge, clinical judgment and reasoning, and patient management and communication. The information provided through the assessment will be useful to licensing boards, hospitals, group practices, managed care organizations, and other health care organizations in making physician licensure and privileging decisions; to identify educational activities needed to enhance a physician's practice patterns; or to assist in career transitions. Assessments may also be beneficial as part of a review of the clinical capabilities of physicians with personal health concerns, such as recovery from disabling illness or injury, neurocognitive concerns, substance abuse, or other issues that may affect practice. Individual physicians may also find assessment services useful in evaluating their clinical competence, particularly if they are at a point of transition in their career or are returning to clinical practice after being away for an extended period of time.

Additional information about the PLAS, its services, and the regional physician evaluation and remediation programs that utilize PLAS assessment resources can be obtained by calling (817) 868-4022 or by visiting the FSMB Web site at *www.fsmb.org*.

Contact Information

Federation of State Medical Boards of the United States, Inc
PO Box 619850
Dallas, TX 75261-9850
(817) 868-4000
(817) 868-4099 Fax
www.fsmb.org

National Board of Medical Examiners® (NBME®)

The National Board of Medical Examiners (NBME) is an independent, not-for-profit organization that provides high-quality examinations for the health professions. Protection of the health of the public through state-of-the-art assessment of health professionals is the mission of the NBME, along with a major commitment to research and development in evaluation and measurement. The NBME was founded in 1915 because of the need for a voluntary, nationwide examination that medical licensing authorities could accept as the standard by which to judge candidates for medical licensure. Since that time, it has continued without interruption to provide high-quality examinations for this purpose and has become a model and a resource of international stature in testing methodologies and evaluation in medicine.

Although the NBME's mission is centered on assessment of physicians, it encompasses the spectrum of health professionals along the continuum of education, training, and practice and includes research in evaluation as well as development of assessment instruments.

United States Medical Licensing Examination® (USMLE®)

The USMLE, cosponsored and co-owned by the NBME and the Federation of State Medical Boards (FSMB), is a three-step examination for medical licensure in the United States. Results of the USMLE are reported to medical licensing authorities in the United States for their use in granting the initial license to practice medicine. The USMLE is the largest NBME examination program. (Information on the USMLE appears on page 86.)

Services for Medical Schools and Health Professional Organizations

Through a liaison program with medical schools, the NBME fosters communication between the NBME and medical schools, and it provides subject tests in the basic and clinical sciences for the purpose of assessing the educational achievement of individuals in specific subject areas. In 2008, the number of subject examinations administered by medical schools was approximately 189,000. The NBME has augmented its subject examination program by implementing a system that allows assembly of customized subject examinations. Customized assessment services were introduced in July 2007 after a final test of the systems that support these services. In 2008, 21 medical schools administered approximately 80 Web-based assessments to 8,390 students.

The NBME also provides testing, educational, consultative, and research services to a number of medical specialty boards, societies, and health sciences organizations. Services include developing, administering, and analyzing examinations for certification, recertification, in-training, self-assessment, or evaluation of special competence. In 2008, the NBME provided services to 27 organizations, including 67 examinations administered to approximately 56,600 examinees.

In 2003, the NBME introduced a Web-based self-assessment program for basic and clinical science content for US and international medical students and graduates. In 2005, the program added a comprehensive clinical medicine self-assessment. For information on these services, visit the NBME Web site at *www.nbme.org*.

Services for the International Community

In 2005, the NBME established an International Programs unit. Its goals include to better protect the health of the US and international public, enhance the quality of health care education throughout the world, contribute to the development of state-of-the-art assessment of health professionals internationally, and have an expanded venue for assessment research activities. Services include test item-writing workshops, item sharing, exam development, consultation services, psychometric consultation, editing, and translations. The NBME and the Foundation for Advancement of International Medical Education and Research (FAIMER®) of the Educational Commission for Foreign Medical Graduates (ECFMG®) collaborate in international medical education initiatives.

Services for Practicing Physicians

The Post-Licensure Assessment System (PLAS) is a joint activity of the NBME and FSMB and was developed to assist medical licensing authorities in assessing physicians who have already been licensed. The PLAS includes the Special Purpose Examination (SPEX®) and the Assessment Center Program. It provides resources for the comprehensive objective and personalized assessments of physicians for whom there is a question regarding clinical competence, such as endorsement of licensure and licensure reactivation after disciplinary action.

Innovation

The NBME continually supports intramural research in the fields of clinical skills assessment, advanced methods of testing, and ongoing studies of the validity and reliability of NBME examination programs. In addition, the Edward J. Stemmler Medical Education Research Fund of the NBME supports medical school research relevant to the mission of the NBME.

The Center for Innovation, with its mission to advance and facilitate the NBME strategic vision through the development of new products and services, implements time-limited pilot projects, researching and applying a range of novel assessment approaches to the full range of medical education and health care needs. A Developmental Programs unit expands projects initiated in the Center for Innovation, moving them toward general use. Its current focus of activities is the continued research and development of an Assessment of Professional Behaviors project.

NBME Certification and Endorsements

The NBME developed and administered its own three-part examination as part of the National Board Certification Program until it was discontinued with the implementation of the USMLE. Certification was awarded to physicians who achieved the following:

- Received the MD degree from an LCME-accredited medical school

- Passed at least one NBME Part or Step examination prior to December 31, 1994 and successfully completed all three Parts/Steps

- Completed, with a satisfactory record, 1 full year (12 months) in a GME program accredited by the Accreditation Council for Graduate Medical Education (accredited internships in Canada were also recognized as meeting this requirement)

Certification by the NBME continues to be used for licensure in the United States for those physicians certified as diplomates prior to implementation of the USMLE and for examinees certified as diplomates who completed a combination of NBME and/or USMLE examinations and passed at least one Part or Step prior to December 31, 1994. The last regular administration of Part I occurred in 1991, Part II in April 1992, and Part III in May 1994. Because some medical students and physicians completed some part of the NBME examination sequence before the implementation of the USMLE, certain combinations of examinations may be considered by medical licensing authorities as comparable to existing examinations. Physicians who passed a combination of examinations should obtain information regarding the acceptability of the combination directly from the medical licensing authority in the jurisdiction where the physician plans to seek licensure.

In 2008, the NBME awarded a total of 24 diplomate certificates, and NBME diplomates requested 6,464 endorsements of certification to medical licensing authorities.

For further information on NBME certification, contact:

NBME
Applicant Services
3750 Market St
Philadelphia, PA 19104
(215) 590-9700

NBME Web Site

Further information on the NBME and its programs and services is available at *www.nbme.org*.

National Board of Osteopathic Medical Examiners (NBOME)

Established in 1934, the National Board of Osteopathic Medical Examiners (NBOME) is a not-for-profit corporation dedicated to serving the public and state licensing agencies by administering examinations testing the medical knowledge and clinical skills of those who seek to practice as osteopathic physicians.

The NBOME examinations have been the primary pathway by which osteopathic physicians have applied for licensure to practice osteopathic medicine. A passing score on the COMLEX-USA sequence verifies a student's adequacy of medical knowledge and clinical skills for practicing osteopathic medicine. Examinations developed by the NBOME are currently accepted in 50 states.

Comprehensive Osteopathic Medical Licensing Examination (COMLEX-USA)

To better assist the state licensing boards in measuring the knowledge required by today's physicians, the NBOME initiated the three-level Comprehensive Osteopathic Medical Licensing Examination (COMLEX-USA) to replace the former three-part NBOME examination series. The COMLEX-USA Level 3 examination was first administered in February 1995, and COMLEX-USA Level 2 was administered for the first time in March 1997. Administration of COMLEX-USA Level 1 in June 1998 completed the transition to COMLEX-USA. Administration of a Performance Evaluation/Clinical Skills component of the COMLEX-USA Level 2, COMLEX-USA Level 2-PE, began in September 2004.

The COMLEX-USA examination series was converted to a computer delivery format with the introduction of Level 2 in July 2005, Level 3 in September 2005, and Level 1 in May 2006.

The COMLEX-USA program is designed to assess the osteopathic medical knowledge and clinical skills considered essential for osteopathic generalist physicians to practice medicine without supervision. COMLEX is constructed in the context of medical problem-solving, which involves clinical presentations and physician tasks.

Candidates are expected to utilize the philosophy and principles of osteopathic medicine to solve medical problems. The Clinical Presentation Dimension identifies high-frequency and/or high-impact health issues that osteopathic generalist physicians commonly encounter in practice. The Physician Task Dimension specifies the major steps osteopathic physicians generally undertake in solving medical problems.

Although all three Levels of COMLEX have the same two-dimensional content structure, the depth and emphases of each Level parallel the educational experiences of the candidates. This progressive nature of the COMLEX program ensures the consistency and continuity of the measurement objectives of osteopathic medical licensing examinations.

Level 1

Level 1 emphasizes the medical concepts and principles necessary for understanding the mechanisms of medical problems and disease processes.

Level 1 is a 1-day, computer-based multiple-choice examination covering the basic medical sciences of anatomy, behavioral science, biochemistry, microbiology, osteopathic principles, pathology, pharmacology, physiology, and other relevant areas.

Level 2-CE (Cognitive Evaluation)

Level 2-CE candidates are expected to demonstrate clinical concepts and principles involved in all steps of medical problem-solving. Level 2 emphasizes the medical concepts and principles necessary for making appropriate medical diagnoses through patient history and physical examination findings.

Level 2-CE is a 1-day, computer-based multiple-choice examination covering the clinical disciplines of community medicine/medical humanities, emergency medicine, internal medicine, obstetrics/gynecology, osteopathic principles, pediatrics, psychiatry, surgery, and other areas necessary to solve medical problems.

Level 2-PE (Performance Evaluation)

COMLEX-USA Level 2-PE is the clinical skills component of the Comprehensive Osteopathic Medical Licensing Examination (COMLEX-USA). Consistent with NBOME's mission to protect the public, COMLEX-USA-Level 2-PE helps to fulfill the public and licensing authority mandate for enhanced patient safety through documentation of the clinical skills proficiency of graduates from osteopathic medical schools.

The COMLEX-USA Level 2-PE is a 1-day examination of clinical skills where each candidate will encounter twelve standardized patients over the course of a 7-hour examination day.

In the Biomedical/Biomechanical Domain of the examination, the candidate is evaluated on data gathering (history and physical diagnosis), osteopathic manipulative skills, and the ability to formulate and legibly write a SOAP note to record the important aspects of the encounter.

The Humanistic Domain requires that the candidate establish the doctor-patient relationship and demonstrate professionalism and the ability to communicate and use interpersonal skills.

Level 3

Level 3 candidates are expected to demonstrate clinical concepts and principles necessary for solving medical problems as independently practicing osteopathic generalist physicians. Level 3 emphasizes the medical concepts and principles required to make appropriate patient management decisions.

Level 3 is a 1-day, computer-based multiple-choice examination covering the clinical disciplines of community medicine/ medical humanities, emergency medicine, internal medicine, obstetrics/gynecology, osteopathic principles, pediatrics, psychiatry, surgery, and other areas necessary to solve medical problems.

Comprehensive Osteopathic Medical Variable-Purpose Examination (COMVEX-USA)

The NBOME offers a post-licensure examination for osteopathic physicians who require reevaluation after initial licensure. The circumstances in which the

Comprehensive Osteopathic Medical Variable-Purpose Examination (COMVEX-USA) may be used include, but are not limited to, the following:

1. An osteopathic physician originally licensed through an examination devoid of osteopathic content is now applying for a license in a state that requires that an osteopathic physician take an osteopathic examination.
2. An osteopathic physician is applying for licensure in a state that imposes a time limit (e.g., completing examination within a 10-year period) and the candidate has not been tested by a licensing board or a certifying board within that time frame.
3. An osteopathic physician is requesting a reinstatement of a license following a career interruption.
4. A tenured osteopathic physician needs to demonstrate basic osteopathic medical competence.

The COMVEX-USA is available in CBT format (previously in paper and pencil format) at professional test centers nationwide (with at least one testing location in each of the 50 states). The examination uses the same basic design features of the COMLEX-USA and employs the same "Dimensions" to assess the candidate. The examination contains 400 test items using objective type questions such as multiple choice, single best answer, and matching test items.

Eligibility for the examination is solely determined by the licensing jurisdiction, and scores are ordinarily returned to the licensing authority within 2 to 3 weeks of the examination date. Licensing boards interested in utilizing this examination may contact the NBOME.

Contact Information

National Board of Osteopathic Medical Examiners, Inc
8765 W Higgins Rd, Ste 200
Chicago, IL 60631-4101
(773) 714-0622
(773) 714-0631 Fax
www.nbome.org

Section IV.

Information for International Medical Graduates

Educational Commission for Foreign Medical Graduates (ECFMG®)

Stephen S. Seeling, JD
Vice President for Operations
Educational Commission for Foreign Medical Graduates
Philadelphia, Pennsylvania

The Educational Commission for Foreign Medical Graduates (ECFMG®), through its program of certification, assesses whether international medical graduates (IMGs) are ready to enter residency or fellowship programs in the United States that are accredited by the Accreditation Council for Graduate Medical Education (ACGME). ECFMG Certification is a requirement for IMGs who wish to enter such programs.

ECFMG Certification assures directors of ACGME-accredited residency and fellowship programs, and the people of the United States, that IMGs have met minimum standards of eligibility to enter such programs. ECFMG Certification does not, however, guarantee that these graduates will be accepted into programs, since the number of applicants exceeds the number of available positions.

ECFMG Certification is also one of the eligibility requirements for IMGs to take Step 3 of the three-step United States Medical Licensing Examination® (USMLE®). Medical licensing authorities in the United States require ECFMG Certification, among other requirements, to obtain an unrestricted license to practice medicine.

The ECFMG and its organizational members define an IMG as a physician who received his/her basic medical degree or qualification from a medical school located outside the United States and Canada. Citizens of the United States who have completed their medical education in schools outside the United States and Canada are considered IMGs; non-US citizens who have graduated from medical schools in the United States and Canada are not considered IMGs.

To be eligible for ECFMG Certification, the physician's medical school and graduation year must be listed in the *International Medical Education Directory* (*IMED*) of the Foundation for Advancement of International Medical Education and Research (FAIMER®). *IMED* contains information supplied by countries about their medical schools. FAIMER is not an accrediting agency. *IMED* is available on the FAIMER Web site at *www.faimer.org*.

ECFMG Examination Requirements

The examination requirements for ECFMG Certification include passing Step 1 and Step 2 of the USMLE. Step 2 has two separately administered components, the Clinical Knowledge (CK) component and the Clinical Skills (CS) component.

To meet the examination requirements for ECFMG Certification, applicants must:

1. Satisfy the Medical Science Examination Requirement. Step 1 and Step 2 CK of the USMLE are the exams currently administered that satisfy this requirement. To meet the medical science examination requirement for ECFMG Certification, applicants must pass both Step 1 and Step 2 CK within a specified period of time. See *Time Limit for Completing Examination Requirements,* on the following page.

Former Examinations Accepted for ECFMG Certification: The ECFMG also accepts a passing performance on the following *former* examinations to satisfy the medical science examination requirement for ECFMG Certification: ECFMG Examination, Visa Qualifying Examination (VQE), Foreign Medical Graduate Examination in the Medical Sciences (FMGEMS), and Part I and Part II Examinations of the National Board of Medical Examiners® (NBME®). Additionally, the ECFMG accepts a score of 75 or higher on each of the 3 days of a single administration of the former Federation Licensing Examination (FLEX), if taken prior to June 1985, to satisfy this requirement.

Combinations of examinations are also acceptable. Specifically, applicants who have passed only part of the former VQE, FMGEMS, or the NBME Part I or Part II may combine a passing performance on the basic medical science component of one of these examinations or USMLE Step 1 with a passing performance on the clinical science component of one of the other examinations or USMLE Step 2 CK, provided that the components are passed within the period specified for the examination program.*

2. Satisfy the Clinical Skills Requirement. Step 2 CS of the USMLE is the exam currently administered that satisfies the clinical skills requirement for ECFMG Certification. Specific time limits for passing Step 2 CS for ECFMG Certification may apply. See *Time Limit for Completing Examination Requirements,* below.

Former Examinations Accepted for ECFMG Certification: Applicants who have *both* passed the former ECFMG Clinical Skills Assessment (CSA®) *and* achieved a score acceptable to ECFMG on an English language proficiency test (such as the Test of English as a Foreign Language™ [TOEFL®] or the former ECFMG English Test) can use these passing performances to satisfy this requirement.

Time Limit for Completing Examination Requirements†

ECFMG policy requires that applicants pass those USMLE Steps and Step Components required for ECFMG Certification within a 7-year period. This means that once an applicant passes a USMLE Step or Step Component, the applicant will have 7 years to pass the other USMLE Step(s) or Step Component(s) required for ECFMG Certification. This 7-year period begins on the exam date for the first Step or Step Component passed and ends *exactly 7 years from this exam date.* If an applicant does

not pass all required USMLE Steps and Step Components within a maximum of 7 years, the applicant's earliest USMLE passing performance will no longer be valid for ECFMG Certification.

This 7-year limit does *not* apply to the former ECFMG CSA because the CSA was not a USMLE Step or Step Component. Applicants who satisfied the clinical skills requirement for ECFMG Certification by passing the CSA are required to pass only Step 1 and Step 2 CK within a 7-year period for ECFMG Certification. For these applicants, the 7-year period begins on the exam date for the first USMLE Step or Step Component passed, regardless of when the CSA was passed.

On June 14, 2004, USMLE Step 2 CS became a requirement for ECFMG Certification, replacing the ECFMG CSA as the exam that satisfies the clinical skills requirement. As part of the USMLE, Step 2 CS may be subject to the 7-year time limit for ECFMG Certification, as described below:

- **If an applicant's earliest USMLE passing performance that is valid for ECFMG Certification took place on or after June 14, 2004,** the applicant is required to pass Step 1, Step 2 CK, and, if required for ECFMG Certification, Step 2 CS within a 7-year period for ECFMG Certification.

- **If an applicant's earliest USMLE passing performance that is valid for ECFMG Certification took place before June 14, 2004,** the applicant is required to pass only Step 1 and Step 2 CK within a 7-year period for ECFMG Certification; if required for ECFMG Certification, Step 2 CS can be passed outside the 7-year period.

*This policy applies only to ECFMG Certification. Use of the former FLEX Components or the former NBME Parts to fulfill eligibility requirements for Step 3 is no longer accepted. Applicants taking the Steps for the purpose of licensure should refer to *Formerly Administered Examinations* in the USMLE *Bulletin of Information.* Applicants should also contact the Federation of State Medical Boards (FSMB) for general information and the medical licensing authority of the jurisdiction where they plan to apply for licensure for definitive information on licensure requirements. Additionally, although the ECFMG Examination and FLEX, if taken prior to June 1985, satisfy the medical science examination requirement for ECFMG Certification, they have not been recognized by the US Secretary of Health and Human Services as meeting the medical science examination requirement to obtain a visa to enter the United States (see *Visas*, page 109).

† These policies apply only to ECFMG Certification. The USMLE program recommends to state medical licensing authorities that they require applicants to pass the full USMLE sequence (including Step 3, which is not required for ECFMG Certification) within a 7-year period. Refer to *Time Limit and Number of Attempts Allowed to Complete All Steps* and *Retakes* in the USMLE *Bulletin of Information.* Applicants should also contact the FSMB for general information and the medical licensing authority of the jurisdiction where they plan to apply for licensure for definitive information, since licensure requirements vary among jurisdictions.

Medical Education Credential Requirements

The physician's medical school and graduation year must be listed in the *International Medical Education Directory* (*IMED*), available on the FAIMER Web site. All IMGs must have had at least 4 credit years (academic years for which credit has been given toward completion of the medical curriculum) in attendance at a medical school listed in *IMED*. There are restrictions on credits transferred to the medical school that awards an applicant's medical degree that can be used to meet this requirement.

Applicants for ECFMG Certification must document the completion of all requirements for, and receipt of, the final medical diploma. ECFMG verifies every applicant's final diploma with the appropriate officials of the medical school that issued the diploma and requests the medical school to provide the applicant's final medical school transcript. Verification by ECFMG with the issuing school may also be required for transcripts that are submitted by applicants to document transferred credits. An applicant's credentials are not considered complete until ECFMG receives and accepts verification of the medical diploma, final medical school transcript, and, if required, transfer credit transcript(s) directly from the issuing school(s).

Standard ECFMG Certificate

The ECFMG issues the Standard ECFMG Certificate to applicants who meet all of the examination and medical education credential requirements. Applicants must also pay any outstanding charges on their ECFMG financial accounts before their certificates are issued. Standard ECFMG Certificates are sent approximately 2 weeks after all of these requirements have been met.

The Standard ECFMG Certificate includes:

- The name of the applicant
- The applicant's USMLE/ECFMG Identification Number
- The dates that examination requirements were met
- The date that the certificate was issued

The Standard ECFMG Certificate may be used for entry into accredited GME programs in the United States.

Important Note: Prior to June 14, 2004, passing performances on an English language proficiency test and the ECFMG Clinical Skills Assessment (CSA) were requirements for ECFMG Certification. Passing performances on these exams were subject to expiration for the purpose of entering US GME programs; Standard ECFMG Certificates based on these exams may list "valid through" dates, the dates through which the passing performances are valid for this purpose. Effective June 14, 2004, some of these examinations are no longer subject to expiration, regardless of whether a "valid through" date is listed on the Standard ECFMG Certificate. See *Validity of Examinations for Entry into GME*, below.

Validity of Examinations for Entry into GME

Clinical Skills Examinations

For applicants who satisfy the clinical skills requirement by passing Step 2 CS, this passing performance is not subject to expiration for the purpose of entering US GME programs.

For applicants who satisfied the clinical skills requirement for ECFMG Certification by passing the former ECFMG CSA and an English language proficiency test, passing performance on the CSA may be subject to expiration for the purpose of entering GME programs, as described below.

- Passing performances on **CSA administrations that took place on or after June 14, 2001**, are not subject to expiration for the purpose of entering GME programs. Applicants who are certified by ECFMG and whose Standard ECFMG Certificate lists a "valid through" date for an administration of the CSA that took place on or after June 14, 2001, may request a permanent validation sticker to be affixed to the certificate. Applicants can request the sticker online by accessing OASIS on the ECFMG Web site.

- Passing performances on **CSA administrations that took place before June 14, 2001**, are valid for 3 years from the date passed for the purpose of entering GME programs. The date through which passing performance on the CSA remains valid for entry into GME (the CSA "valid through" date) will be listed on the applicant's Standard ECFMG Certificate. If the applicant entered a program before expiration of the valid through date, the applicant may request permanent validation. This means

Table 29

Examinee Performance for International Medical Graduates/Students Taking USMLE Step 1 and Step 2 (CK and CS) Examinations

	USMLE Step 1 January 1, 2008 - December 31, 2008			USMLE Step 2 CK July 1, 2007 - June 30, 2008			USMLE Step 2 CS July 1, 2007 - June 30, 2008		
	Number of Administrations	Number Passing	Percent Passing	Number of Administrations	Number Passing	Percent Passing	Number of Administrations	Number Passing	Percent Passing
Total	**20,387**	**12,835**	**63**	**16,170**	**12,036**	**74**	**17,231**	**12,060**	**70**
First-time Takers	14,850	10,790	73	12,847	10,358	81	13,748	9,836	72
Repeaters	5,537	2,045	37	3,323	1,678	50	3,483	2,224	64
US Citizens	**5,194**	**2,734**	**53**	**3,431**	**2,167**	**63**	**3,185**	**2,531**	**79**
First-time Takers	3,119	2,096	67	2,337	1,664	71	2,689	2,181	81
Repeaters	2,075	638	31	1,094	503	46	496	350	71
Foreign Citizens	**15,193**	**10,101**	**66**	**12,739**	**9,869**	**77**	**14,046**	**9,529**	**68**
First-time Takers	11,731	8,694	74	10,510	8,694	83	11,059	7,655	69
Repeaters	3,462	1,407	41	2,229	1,175	53	2,987	1,874	63

Notes: Step 1 first-time takers are those examinees with no prior Step 1 and no prior NBME Part I examinations.

Step 2 CK first-time takers are those examinees with no prior Step 2 CK and no prior NBME Part II examinations.

Step 2 CS first-time takers are those examinees with no prior Step 2 CS and no prior ECFMG CSA examinations.

Administrations include those with results of Pass, Fail, Incomplete, Indeterminate, and Withheld.

The data for repeaters represents examinations given, not examinees.

Citizenship is as of the time of entrance into medical school.

Source: ECFMG database. Data current as of February 5, 2009, and include administrations for which results were available as of February 4, 2009.

that the CSA date is no longer subject to expiration. To request permanent validation, the applicant and an authorized official of the training institution must complete a *Request for Permanent Validation* (Form 246), available on the ECFMG Web site. On receipt of this form, ECFMG will provide a permanent validation sticker to be affixed to the certificate. If an applicant who passed CSA before June 14, 2001, did not enter a GME program within 3 years of the CSA pass date, the applicant's CSA passing performance has expired for the purpose of entering GME. Before entering a program, these applicants must pass Step 2 CS. Passing performance on Step 2 CS does not expire for the purpose of entry into GME.

English Examinations

Passing performances on the English language proficiency test formerly required by ECFMG (such as the TOEFL exam or the former ECFMG English Test) are not subject to expiration for the purpose of entering GME programs, regardless of the date passed. Applicants who are certified by ECFMG and whose Standard ECFMG Certificate lists a "valid through" date for an English language proficiency test may request a permanent validation sticker to be

affixed to the certificate. Applicants can request the sticker online by accessing OASIS on the ECFMG Web site.

Important Note: The preceding discussion of validity and expiration of examinations, and the "valid through" and "valid indefinitely" designations on the Standard ECFMG Certificate (if applicable), are relevant *only* for the purpose of entry into US GME programs. They do *not* pertain to eligibility for USMLE Step 3 or to any time limits imposed by medical licensing authorities or other entities for the completion of all USMLE Steps.

Step 1 and Step 2 of the USMLE

The USMLE is a three-step examination for medical licensure in the United States that provides a common system to evaluate applicants for medical licensure. The USMLE is sponsored by the FSMB and the NBME. The USMLE is governed by a committee consisting of members of the FSMB, NBME, ECFMG, and the American public. The USMLE Steps 1, 2, and 3 replaced FLEX and the NBME Parts I, II, and III.

Table 30
Standard ECFMG Certificates Issued in 2008: Distribution of Recipients by Country of Medical School and Citizenship

Country	Country of Medical School		Country of Citizenship	
	Number	%	Number	%
Australia	65	0.6	44	0.4
Bangladesh	59	0.6	49	0.5
Brazil	97	0.9	99	1.0
Canada	0	0.0	276	2.7
Cayman Islands	131	1.3	0	0.0
China	322	3.1	323	3.1
Colombia	132	1.3	133	1.3
Cuba	58	0.6	66	0.6
Dominica	696	6.8	6	<0.1
Dominican Republic	138	1.3	68	0.7
Egypt	206	2.0	184	1.8
Germany	120	1.2	93	0.9
Greece	51	0.5	48	0.5
Grenada	540	5.3	4	<0.1
India	2,637	25.7	2,695	26.2
Iran	174	1.7	189	1.8
Iraq	60	0.6	56	0.5
Ireland	124	1.2	67	0.7
Israel	151	1.5	75	0.7
Japan	56	0.5	55	0.5
Jordan	105	1.0	118	1.1
Lebanon	125	1.2	135	1.3
Mexico	121	1.2	72	0.7
Nepal	157	1.5	166	1.6
Netherlands Antilles	407	4.0	0	0.0
Nigeria	199	1.9	207	2.0
Pakistan	654	6.4	618	6.0
Peru	75	0.7	82	0.8
Philippines	370	3.6	330	3.2
Poland	113	1.1	32	0.3
Romania	107	1.0	94	0.9
Russia	124	1.2	71	0.7
Saint Kitts and Nevis	103	1.0	3	<0.1
South Korea	103	1.0	108	1.1
Syria	168	1.6	164	1.6
Turkey	57	0.6	50	0.5
Ukraine	75	0.7	51	0.5
United Kingdom	82	0.8	112	1.1
United States	0	0.0	2,064	20.1
Venezuela	58	0.6	56	0.5
Countries with fewer than 50 recipients	1,255	12.2	1,212	11.8
Total	**10,275**	**100.0**	**10,275**	**100.0**

Notes: Citizenship is as of the time of entrance into medical school.

Percentages may not equal 100% due to rounding.

Data current as of January 9, 2009.

The ECFMG determines whether international medical students/graduates are eligible to take USMLE Step 1 and Step 2 and registers eligible applicants to take these exams for the purpose of ECFMG Certification. The NBME registers eligible students/graduates of US and Canadian medical schools/programs accredited by the Liaison Committee on Medical Education or the American Osteopathic Association to take Step 1 and Step 2.

USMLE Step 1 and Step 2 CK are multiple-choice examinations that are administered by computer. Prometric™ provides scheduling and test centers for Step 1 and Step 2 CK. These exams are delivered throughout the year at Prometric test centers worldwide.

Step 2 CS uses standardized patients in simulated clinical encounters to evaluate clinical and communication skills. Step 2 CS is administered throughout the year at test centers in Atlanta, Chicago, Houston, Los Angeles, and Philadelphia.

Table 29 shows the performance of IMGs for recent administrations of Step 1 and Step 2 (CK and CS).

Standard ECFMG Certificates Issued in 2008

During 2008, 10,275 Standard ECFMG Certificates were issued. Table 30 shows the distribution of recipients of Standard ECFMG Certificates by country of medical school and citizenship. In 2008, medical schools in India and Dominica had the largest number of recipients: 2,637 (25.7%) and 696 (6.8%), respectively.

Based upon country of citizenship, citizens of India formed the largest group of recipients. Of the certificates issued in 2008, 2,695 (26.2%) were to Indian citizens. Citizens of the United States were the second largest group with 2,064 (20.1%) recipients.

Electronic Residency Application Service (ERAS®)

The Association of American Medical Colleges (AAMC) developed the Electronic Residency Application Service (ERAS®) to allow Web-based application to residency programs. ECFMG serves as the designated Dean's office for students and graduates of international medical schools, including Fifth Pathway participants, who use ERAS. In this role, ECFMG assists these individuals with the ERAS application process for first- and second-year residency positions. This includes transmitting applicants' supporting documents, reports of ECFMG certification status, and, if requested by the applicant, USMLE transcripts to the ERAS PostOffice, where they are available for downloading by residency programs to which applicants have applied.

Most medical specialties participate in ERAS. Programs in participating specialties require applicants to apply for positions using ERAS.

For a list of specialties participating in ERAS for residency programs that begin in 2010, visit *http://services.aamc.org/eras/erasstats/par/*

Additional specialties may use ERAS for residency programs that begin in 2011. Applicants should contact residency program directors for specific requirements and deadlines.

For information, visit the ECFMG Web site at *www.ecfmg.org/eras*. Applicants may also contact:

ERAS Support Services at
ECFMG
3624 Market St
Philadelphia, PA 19104-2685
E-mail: *eras-support@ecfmg.org*
(215) 386-5900

Visas

To obtain a visa to enter the United States to perform services as members of the medical profession or to receive GME, certain foreign national physicians are required, under the provisions of Public Law 94-484, to pass the NBME Part I and Part II examinations or an examination determined to be equivalent for this purpose. The Secretary of Health and Human Services has recognized USMLE Step 1 and Step 2 as well as the former Visa Qualifying Examination (VQE) and the Foreign Medical Graduate Examination in the Medical Sciences (FMGEMS) as equivalent to NBME Part I and Part II examinations for the purposes of PL 94-484. To obtain additional information on visa requirements, foreign national physicians should refer to the following Web sites:

- ECFMG Exchange Visitor Sponsorship Program *www.ecfmg.org/evsp*
- US Embassies or Consulates of the US Department of State (DOS) *www.usembassy.gov*
- Immigration Bureaus of the US Department of Homeland Security (DHS) *www.dhs.gov*

Exchange Visitor Sponsorship Program

The ECFMG is authorized by the United States Department of State (DOS) to sponsor foreign national physicians as J-1 Exchange Visitors in GME or training programs. The objectives of this program are to enhance international exchange in the field of medicine and to promote mutual understanding between the people of the United States and other countries through the interchange of persons, knowledge, and skills.

Table 31
Exchange Visitor Sponsorship Program for Physicians: Number of J-1 Physicians in Graduate Medical Education or Training Programs in the United States, 2007-2008 Academic Year

Specialty	Count
Allergy and Immunology	8
Anesthesiology	88
Colon and Rectal Surgery	13
Dermatology	20
Emergency Medicine	49
Family Medicine	503
Internal Medicine	2,884
Internal Medicine/Family Medicine	1
Internal Medicine/Medical Genetics	1
Internal Medicine/Neurology	1
Internal Medicine/Pediatrics	36
Internal Medicine/Preventive Medicine	4
Internal Medicine/Psychiatry	11
Medical Genetics	11
Medical Genetics and Pathology	3
Neurological Surgery	56
Neurology	236
Nuclear Medicine	12
Obstetrics and Gynecology	179
Ophthalmology	40
Orthopaedic Surgery	91
Otolaryngology	39
Pathology - Anatomic and Clinical	163
Pediatrics	675
Pediatrics/Medical Genetics	3
Physical Medicine and Rehabilitation	23
Plastic Surgery	19
Preventive Medicine (General, Public Health, Occupational Medicine, Aerospace Medicine)	1
Psychiatry	369
Radiation Oncology	6
Radiology - Diagnostic	86
Sleep Medicine	5
Surgery - General	486
Thoracic Surgery	67
Transitional Year	15
Urology	31
Total	**6,235**

The program is administered by ECFMG in accordance with the provisions set forth in an agreement between the ECFMG and the DOS and the federal regulations established to implement the Mutual Educational and Cultural Exchange Act. The ECFMG is responsible for ensuring that all Exchange Visitor Physicians and host institutions comply with the federal requirements for participation. The ECFMG issues a Certificate of Eligibility

for Exchange Visitor (J-1) Status (Form DS-2019) for qualified applicants. This document must be processed through the United States Embassy or Consulate of the US DOS and/or the immigration bureaus of the US DHS.

The federal regulations refer to Exchange Visitor Physicians seeking J-1 sponsorship in clinical programs as *alien physicians.* These applicants must meet, among other requirements, a number of general requirements, which are detailed in the ECFMG's application materials for J-1 visa sponsorship. At a minimum, applicants must:

- Have passed USMLE Step 1 and Step 2 CK; or the former VQE, NBME Part I and Part II, or FMGEMS examinations; or an acceptable combination thereof. (*Note:* The former 1-day ECFMG Examination and FLEX do not meet the requirements for J-1 visa sponsorship.)

- Hold a Standard ECFMG Certificate without expired examination dates, if applicable. *Note:* See *Validity of Examinations for Entry into GME*, page 106, for important information. (Graduates of LCME- and AOA-accredited US and Canadian medical schools/programs are not required to be ECFMG-certified.)

- Hold a contract or an official letter of offer for a position in an approved GME or training program.

- Provide a statement of need from the Ministry of Health of the country of most recent legal permanent residence. This statement must provide written assurance that the country needs specialists in the area in which the Exchange Visitor will receive training. It also serves to confirm the physician's commitment to return to that country upon completion of training in the United States. (*Note:* If permanent residence is in a country other than that of citizenship, the Ministry of Health letter must come from the country of most recent legal permanent residence.)

The duration of stay for a J-1 Exchange Visitor physician is limited to the time typically required to complete the advanced medical education program. This refers to the specialty and subspecialty certification requirements published by the American Board of Medical Specialties (ABMS®). Participation is further limited to 7 years and is reserved for those progressing in approved training programs.

J-1 Exchange Visitor Physicians sponsored for participation in nonclinical programs primarily involved with observation, consultation, teaching, or research are categorized as *research scholars.* Unlike alien physicians, participants in these programs are not required to be ECFMG-certified. Research scholars are limited to activities involving no patient contact or only incidental patient contact. The maximum period of participation for research scholars is 5 years.

Table 31 shows that the ECFMG sponsored 6,235 Exchange Visitor Physicians in US GME or training programs for the 2007-2008 academic year. In the alien physician category, the ECFMG sponsored 4,461 in clinical residency (specialty) programs and 1,712 in clinical fellowships (subspecialty training) in 2007-2008. A total of 62 foreign nationals were sponsored in the research scholar category. Foreign nationals from India, Canada, and Pakistan represented approximately one third of ECFMG-sponsored J-1 physicians for this period.

For application materials and specific information on ECFMG sponsorship, applicants should visit the ECFMG Web site at *www.ecfmg.org/evsp*. Applicants may also contact:

ECFMG
Exchange Visitor Sponsorship Program
3624 Market St
Philadelphia, PA 19104-2685
(215) 823-2121
(215) 386-9766 Fax

Certification Verification Service (CVS)

The ECFMG's Certification Verification Service provides primary-source confirmation of the ECFMG certification status of IMGs. The Joint Commission, the organization that evaluates and accredits US health care organizations and programs, has determined that direct verification with ECFMG of a physician's certification status satisfies The Joint Commission's requirement for primary-source verification of medical school completion for IMGs.

The ECFMG will confirm an applicant's certification status when a request is received from a medical licensing authority, residency program director, hospital, or other organization that, in the judgment of ECFMG, has a legitimate interest in such information. For status reports sent to medical licensing authorities, the request can also be made by the applicant. Requesting organizations must normally secure and retain the applicant's signed authorization to obtain certification information. Please note that there may be a fee for this service.

Requests for confirmation must contain the applicant's name, date of birth, and USMLE/ECFMG Identification Number, as well as the name and address of the organization to which the confirmation should be sent. Confirmations are sent to the requesting organization within approximately 2 weeks. Confirmations are not sent to applicants directly.

For individuals who apply to residency programs through ERAS, the ECFMG automatically sends an electronic ECFMG status report to the ERAS PostOffice, where it can be accessed by residency programs.

If an applicant's ECFMG certification status changes during the ERAS application process, the ECFMG will automatically send an updated status report to the ERAS PostOffice.

To obtain information, request form(s), or make an online request, refer to the CVS home page on the ECFMG Web site at *www.ecfmg.org/cvs* or contact:

ECFMG
CVS Department
PO Box 13679
Philadelphia PA 19101-3679
(215) 386-5900

Contact Information

Interested individuals can access the ECFMG *Information Booklet* and apply online for USMLE Step 1 and Step 2 by visiting the ECFMG Web site at *www.ecfmg.org*. The ECFMG Web site also provides access to important updates, ECFMG's online services, and more than 50 ECFMG publications and forms.

Individuals who do not have access to the Internet may contact the ECFMG for assistance.

ECFMG
3624 Market St
Philadelphia, PA 19104-2685
(215) 386-5900
(215) 386-9196 Fax
E-mail: *info@ecfmg.org*
www.ecfmg.org

Immigration Overview for International Medical Graduates

Robert D. Aronson, partner
Aronson & Associates, PA, Minneapolis, Minnesota

This article outlines current immigration laws and policies that affect the physician community. This particular legal area has become increasingly important owing to the emerging shortage of physicians in the workforce and the maldistribution patterns largely affecting rural and inner city communities. As a result of the inability of domestic physicians to satisfy these emerging needs, there have been a number of new initiatives of particular relevance to the immigration of international medical graduates (IMGs).

This article deals with three broad areas of relevance to the immigration of IMGs:

1. Temporary, nonimmigrant visa options for foreign physicians
2. The J-1 waiver process for physicians
3. Options in order to qualify for permanent residence

Immigration Law Overview

All foreign nationals enter the United States in one of two broad immigration categories—either under a temporary, nonimmigrant visa or as a permanent resident. There are comparative advantages to both these categories. In the case of the temporary, nonimmigrant visa classifications, it is usually possible to gain this type of immigration coverage in a relatively short time. The two most commonly used temporary, nonimmigrant classifications by IMGs are the J-1 Exchange Visitor program and the H-1B Temporary Worker classification. Both these classifications, however, limit a physician's duration of residence in the United States and impose strict limitations on the range of employment authorization, although they do have the advantage of being relatively quick to obtain. In contrast, permanent residence provides a foreign national with both an unlimited duration of residence and full, unrestricted employment authorization, although the processing time is much greater.

Temporary, Nonimmigrant Classifications

Most IMGs in graduate medical education (GME) programs arrive under the J-1 Exchange Visitor program, although the H-1B Temporary Worker category is becoming increasingly utilized.

The J-1 program is administered by the Educational Commission for Foreign Medical Graduates (ECFMG), working under the authorization of the US Department of State. J-1 training programs are intended to provide a broad range of foreign nationals with educational, employment, and training opportunities in the United States. For the past 30 years, the J-1 Exchange Visitor Program has been the preferred visa classification for IMGs doing their medical training in the United States.

To become eligibile to enroll in GME, an IMG needs to establish that his/her medical competency is equivalent to that of a US physician. This professional equivalency is established through the issuance of ECFMG certification. To gain an ECFMG Certificate, an IMG needs to fulfill the following requirements:

1. Pass stipulated examinations—currently, the US Medical Licensing Examination (USMLE), Steps 1 and 2 Clinical Knowledge and Clinical Skills—to establish medical competence and English language competence

2. Pass the ECFMG English language examination to establish English language competence

3. Possess an MD degree from a foreign medical school listed in the *International Medical Education Directory* of the Foundation for Advancement of International Medical Education and Research (FAIMER®)

All J-1 trainees must receive ECFMG certification, except for graduates of Canadian medical schools, who are exempt from this requirement because Canadian medical education and training are accredited under US standards (or considered equivalent to US education/training).

Upon entry into the United States, an IMG is authorized to pursue a clinical GME program for up to 7 years to achieve stipulated training objectives. Each year, the GME program, in conjunction with the IMG, needs to file an extension application with the ECFMG.

Without exception, all J-1 physicians engaged in clinical training activities are subject to a mandatory 2-year home residence obligation, regardless of country of citizenship or last permanent residence. *Note:* This 2-year home residence requirement applies to every physician who enters the United States under an ECFMG-sponsored J-1 clinical training program. To ultimately qualify for permanent residence and/or an H-1B visa, an IMG must either return to his/her home country for a 2-year period or obtain a waiver of this 2-year obligation.

J-1 Waiver Strategies

As noted above, all ECFMG-sponsored J-1 physicians—regardless of country of citizenship—are subject to an obligation to return to their home country for a mandatory 2-year period. Unless and until this 2-year home residence is either fulfilled (i.e., by returning specifically to the home country) or waived (i.e., eliminated), a physician under law is barred from obtaining an H-1B visa and/or permanent resident status. Therefore, it is critically important for long-term immigration prospects for a J-1 physician to obtain a waiver of the 2-year home residence requirement. US laws do contain various provisions enabling J-1 physicians to obtain such waivers.

A waiver of this obligation is available only on the basis of at least one the following three grounds:

- If the J-1 physician will suffer from persecution in his/her home country or country of last permanent residence

- If fulfillment of the obligation will subject a US citizen spouse or child to exceptional hardship

- Based upon a recommendation issued by a government agency interested in the physician's continued residence/employment in the United States

Without question, the vast majority of J-1 physicians who receive waivers do so through recommendations issued by government agencies. Generally speaking, such waivers fall within the following three basic patterns:

- Employment by a federal agency, such as the Department of Veterans Affairs

- Recognition of outstanding academic and research achievements, as determined by the Department of Health and Human Services

- Service to medically underserved patient populations, so as to allow either a state department of health or a federal agency to recommend a waiver as a matter of public interest

Statistically, the vast majority of J-1 physicians have obtained waivers through a program known as the Conrad State 30 program, which essentially empowers each state to recommend waivers for up to 30 physicians per fiscal year. These waivers specifically require the physician to practice medicine (either primary care or specialty) in a designated medically underserved location.

Most states now recommend waivers for medical specialists as well as primary care practitioners. Although each state is limited to 30 waivers/year, a state now has the option of using up to 10 waivers/year to facilitate placements in non-medically underserved areas. The remaining balance can only be used for placements in designated medically underserved areas—i.e., Health Professional Shortage Areas (HPSAs) or Medically Underserved Areas/Populations (MUA/Ps). In any case, the key point is to show that the physician will be serving the needs of the indigent and medically underserved—i.e., patient populations that disproportionately face barriers in their access to physicians. A physician receiving a J-1 waiver needs to practice medicine in the community for at least 3 years, working specifically in H-1B status. Any premature departure from the community could result in a loss of the waiver as well as immigration status.

While the Conrad waiver program will sunset on September 30, 2009, it has been a widely used program for recruitment and retention of physicians in traditionally underserved communities. It is expected that this program will continue to be extended and, quite possibly, enlarged.

In addition, various federal agencies also maintain J-1 waiver programs, including the Department of Health and Human Services, Delta Regional Commission, and Appalachian Regional Commission. Most federal agencies, however, limit their waiver programs to primary care physicians, even though the law was liberalized in December 2004 to cover medical specialists. The federal agencies do not, though, have any quota limitation on the number of waivers that they can recommend.

H1-B Temporary Worker

Instead of taking part in the J-1 Exchange Visitor program, with its home residence obligation, an increasing number of foreign physicians are entering the United States under the H-1B Temporary Worker provisions. This visa classification enables a foreign national to enter the United States for professional-level employment for up to 6 years. In most instances, H-1B coverage can be obtained within approximately 60-90 days, although there are provisions for expediting the processing of an immigration case. The H-1B quota of 65,000 is normally exhausted early on in the federal fiscal year, but physicians working within universities and most university-affiliated institutions as well as J-1 physicians holding waivers are exempted from the H-1B quota.

To qualify for H-1B benefits, an IMG must meet the following four criteria:

- Possession of a full, unrestricted state medical license or the "appropriate authorization" for the position

- An MD degree or a full, unrestricted foreign license

- English language competence as established either through graduation from an accredited medical school or by holding an ECFMG Certificate

- Passage of the Federation Licensing Examination (FLEX) or its equivalents—the National Board of Medical Examiners (NBME), Parts I, II, and III, or the USMLE, Steps 1, 2, and 3

As a result of the FLEX equivalency issue, many Canadian physicians do not qualify for H-1B benefits. The standard Canadian medical credential—the Licentiate of the Medical Council of Canada (LMCC)—is widely accepted among the states for medical licensure purposes. Therefore, most Canadian physicians have traditionally not had any reason to sit for the FLEX or its equivalents. Over the course of recent years, a significant number of Canadian physicians have begun sitting for the USMLE precisely to gain H-1B eligibility as a clinical physician in the United States.

Permanent Residence Strategies

A foreign national can qualify for permanent residence in various ways, ranging from familial relationships with US citizens or permanent residents to fear of persecution that would merit refugee entitlement. In most instances, though, an IMG will need to qualify for permanent residence based upon an employment position. There are three basic pathways to permanent residence based upon employment as a physician.

Pathway One

The "normal" route to permanent residence involves a three-step process. The first and arguably most complex stage is the Labor Certification Application process. This is a procedure conducted under the auspices of the US Department of Labor to establish that the employment of a foreign national will in no manner harm the US labor market, particularly by taking a job away from a fully qualified US worker. Therefore, acting under a complex recruitment/advertisement procedure, the employer needs to show that the IMG is not simply the best-qualified applicant for the position but is the only fully qualified candidate for the specific position. Effective March 28, 2005, the Labor Certification Application process was reengineered into the PERM Program, which places certain constraints on this process but speeds up considerably the processing time for such applications.

After completing the Labor Certification Application process, the employer needs to submit an Immigrant Visa Petition to the US Citizenship and Immigration Services (CIS, formerly the Immigration and Naturalization Service), establishing the complete suitability of the IMG for the position. Upon approval of this petition, the IMG is then able to actually apply for permanent residence either through a CIS District Office (adjustment of status) or through a US Consular post (consular processing).

Note: An IMG must possess an ECFMG Certificate. Also, an IMG cannot finalize the application for permanent residence status if he/she has an unfulfilled or unwaived J-1 2-year home residence obligation.

Pathway Two

A second pathway to employment-related permanent residence is based upon National Interest Waiver criteria. In this instance, an IMG has a streamlined, expedited pathway to permanent residence if it can be shown that the IMG's employment as a physician carries potential major benefits to areas of high national interest. Under recent revisions to the law, both primary and specialty care physicians working in designated medically underserved areas can qualify for permanent residence pursuant to a National Interest Waiver. Any physician using this pathway, however, has an obligation of working in a designated medically underserved community for a minimum of five years.

Pathway Three

A third option to permanent residence is available to physicians of extraordinarily high professional capabilities, working either in clinical practice or in academic medicine. Such individuals may qualify for permanent residence under an expedited procedure established for Aliens of Extraordinary Ability and Outstanding Professors or Researchers.

Final Word

In conclusion, our immigration laws for physicians are complex, but with advance planning, it is often quite possible to attain desired immigration objectives in a time-efficient manner. Slowly but surely, our immigration laws and policies are creating some new opportunities that enable IMGs to attain immigration status based on practice in the profession, particularly if working in designated medically underserved areas. When all is said and done, we as a nation have complex and ever-expanding needs for physicians, particularly those willing to serve in isolated areas and those willing to treat minorities, ethnic populations, and the indigent. Over the years, foreign physicians have been one of the most effective physician population groups for addressing medically underserved populations, and our immigration laws have developed several meaningful and effective initiatives intended to facilitate the relocation of foreign physicians into positions of maximum benefit to various US population groups.

Robert D. Aronson is the managing partner for Aronson & Associates, PA, a law firm that practices exclusively in the area of immigration and nationality law. The major area of his practice deals with immigration matters for foreign physicians and US medical institutions nationwide. He received his law degree from Indiana University and was a Fulbright Fellow at Harvard Law School and Moscow State University (Russia). Mr. Aronson has held various leadership positions on immigration matters for international physicians within the medical, legal, academic, and governmental communities. Further information is available at www.aronsonimmigration.com.

Section V.

Federal and National Programs and Activities

Licensure in the US Armed Forces

Department of the Air Force

Dale R. Agner, Col, USAF, MC
Chief, Clinical Quality Management Division

Kathy A. Smith, CPHQ, CPCS, CPMSM
Chief, Professional Staff Management
Air Force Medical Operations Agency/SGHQ
Office of the Surgeon General
San Antonio, Texas

The Clinical Quality Management Division of the Air Force Medical Operations Agency is responsible for oversight of clinical issues pertaining to quality improvement, licensure, credentialing and privileging, patient safety, and risk management for the Air Force Surgeon General.

Air Force licensure policy is consistent with that of the Department of Defense (DoD). Air Force Medical Service physicians (military, civil service, contract personnel, and volunteers) must possess a current, valid, and unrestricted license from an official agency of a state; the District of Columbia; or a commonwealth, territory, or possession of the United States to provide health care independently within the scope of the license. Physicians must have a medical license that meets all clinical, professional, and administrative requirements of the issuing state and be no different than that of civilian counterparts.

Personnel accessed from professional training or who complete other training and require a license must obtain such license within 1 year of the date when all required didactic and clinical requirements are met, or within 1 year of completion of graduate year one. Physicians who do not yet meet licensure requirements may practice only under a written plan of supervision by a licensed, fully qualified, independently practicing, privileged provider of same or similar specialty. The Air Force requires physicians who choose to be licensed in a state that requires more than 1 year of graduate training to first obtain a license from a state that requires only 1 year of graduate training.

Department of the Army

Howard M. Kimes, Colonel, US Army
Director, Quality Management Directorate

Janet L. Wilson, Lieutenant Colonel, US Army
Chief, Regulatory Compliance
US Army Medical Command
Fort Sam Houston, Texas

The US Army Medical Command's Quality Management Directorate is responsible for developing policy and overseeing all facets of the Army Surgeon General's Quality Assurance Program, including quality improvement, credentials review and privileging, licensure, and risk management. The Directorate serves as the conduit for issues concerning clinical standards and accreditation by The Joint Commission for US Army Medicine Worldwide.

Department of Defense physicians (military and civilian, contractors and partners) must possess a current valid, unrestricted license from an official agency of the District of Columbia or a state, commonwealth, territory, or possession of the United States to provide health care independently within the scope of their licenses. Physicians in graduate medical education (GME) programs must possess a license within 1 year from the completion of their first year of GME training. An exception exists for individuals who complete their first year of GME in a state requiring 2 or more years of GME for licensure and who are assigned with that same state. These individuals must possess a license within 1 year of completion of their second year of GME training.

Health care providers awaiting a required license work only under the supervision of a licensed provider.

Department of the Navy

Joseph McBreen, Captain,
Medical Corps, US Navy
Director, Clinical Operations
Bureau of Medicine and Surgery
Department of the Navy
Washington, DC

Georgi Irvine, Commander, NC, US (Ret), BSN, MA,
CPHQ, CLNC
Head, Medical and Dental Staff Services
Navy Medical Support Command
Jacksonville, Florida

The Clinical Operations Division within the Bureau of Medicine and Surgery, Department of the Navy (DON), is responsible for developing policy and directing the development and implementation of US Navy-wide quality management and professional affairs programs to improve the quality of patient care; reduce risks to our customers, guests, and staff; advance good stewardship; and maintain accreditation by The Joint Commission of all US Navy fixed medical treatment facilities.

Federal regulations require physicians and other health providers within the military health services system to possess a professional license or certification. The DON further requires the license to be current, valid, unrestricted, and one to which quality management data accrues. All DON physicians (military, civilian, civilian contract, and partnership), except interns, must possess a license from a recognized, official agency of a state; the District of Columbia; or a commonwealth, territory, or possession of the United States to provide health care services independently within the scope of their license. Licenses issued by authorities allowing reduced or no fees for military personnel must meet the same licensure criteria. Health care practitioners lacking required license or certification may work only under a plan of supervision with a licensed practitioner of the same or a similar professional discipline. This policy supports the US Navy's goal to ensure all practitioners are available for worldwide assignment and rapid deployment.

Federal Controlled Substances Registration

Office of Diversion Control
Drug Enforcement Administration
Washington, DC

The Controlled Substances Act of 1970 mandates that controlled substances be maintained in a "closed system of distribution" that tracks all phases of manufacture, distribution, and dispensing. The Department of Justice, through the Drug Enforcement Administration (DEA), has the responsibility to ensure the availability of controlled substances for legitimate need while preventing their diversion into illicit markets.

The Controlled Substances Act and its implementing regulations require that any person desiring to legally manufacture, distribute, or dispense controlled substances must register with the DEA. After approval, each applicant is assigned a registration number, which must be used in every transaction involving controlled substances. Use of the DEA registration number, together with required records of transactions, allows tracking of controlled substances from the point of manufacture to the point at which they are dispensed to the patient.

As of April 20, 2009, there were 1,328,064 active DEA registrants. Practitioners account for 1,032,151of those registrants.

A physician who seeks to become registered with the DEA must submit an Application for Registration (DEA Form-224). There are several means of submitting an application.

A. Online Application Form

Application forms are available on the DEA Diversion Control Program Web site at *www.DEAdiversion.usdoj.gov*. Both the new application (DEA Form-224) and the renewal form (DEA Form-224a) may be completed online in one of the following ways:

1. Applications may be completed and submitted via DEA's "Office of Diversion Control Web Interactive Forms (ODWIF)." Physicians will need a browser that supports 128-bit encryption, and they must have their Tax ID and/or Social Security Number; State Controlled Substance Registration Information; State Medical License Information; and a credit card (American Express, Discover, Visa, or MasterCard) to complete the transaction. This transaction takes approximately 5 minutes and is transmitted to DEA HQ in a secure and encrypted manner.

2. Applications may be also completed in a partially interactive form in Adobe Acrobat PDF format online, where the registrant fills in the information then prints, signs, and mails the printed form to the below address.

3. Blank applications may be printed from the DEA's Web site and then filled out manually by the registrant, signed, and mailed to the below address.

B. Paper Application Form

The form can be obtained from DEA by calling the Registration Unit at (800) 882-9539 or contacting a DEA field office with a registration assistant. The completed paper application (DEA Form-224) and the required fee must be mailed to:

Drug Enforcement Administration
Central Station
PO Box 530295
Atlanta, GA 30348-0295

Following initial processing by the Registration Unit, the application is referred to the appropriate DEA field office for completion after verification of controlled substances authority with the state. The application is approved and a certificate bearing the practitioner's DEA registration number is issued. This process normally takes from 4 to 6 weeks to complete. (Renewal applications generally are processed within 4 weeks.) The online new application takes approximately 5 days till a registration certification is mailed. If there are no changes from the previous registration, online renewals are mailed the following day. The DEA certificate must be maintained at the registered location and must be kept available for official inspection.

The DEA also registers practitioners who have been granted limited authority by the appropriate state licensing agency to handle controlled substances. These individuals are registered as mid-level practitioners (MLPs). As of April 20, 2009, 161,833 mid-level practitioners, including nurse practitioners, certified nurse-midwives, physician assistants, and optometrists, were registered with DEA.

The fee for both new and renewal applications for all practitioners is currently $551 for a 3-year period. An exemption from payment of the application fee is provided to federal, state, or local government registrants. On August 29, 2006, the DEA published a Final Rule in the *Federal Register* (Volume 71, Number 167, pages 51105-51115) that increased the fee to $551 for a 3-year period. The fee schedule is effective for all new and renewal applications postmarked on or after November 1, 2006.

A renewal application, DEA Form 224a, is mailed to each registrant approximately 60 days prior to the expiration date. Registrants who do not receive the form within 45 days prior to the expiration of their registration should contact a DEA office with a registration assistant to request a renewal application. DEA registrations are issued for controlled substances activities at specific locations. If a physician has more than one office where controlled substances will be stored, a separate registration must be obtained for each location. If the activities at a secondary location are limited to prescribing within the same state, then separate registration is not required.

The following registration information is provided:

1. When submitting a new or renewal application, or requesting a modification of a registration, allow 4 weeks for processing; DEA receives more than 35,000 requests per month.

2. One of the primary criteria for issuing a DEA registration is that the applicant be authorized by the state in which he or she will practice. Make sure that all applications for state licensing have been completed before submitting your application for DEA registration. The same applies for registrants relocating from one state to another.

3. Keep track of the expiration date of your DEA registration. Renewal notices are mailed to registrants approximately 60 days prior to expiration. If you do not receive a renewal application within 45 days prior to the expiration of your registration, call (800) 882-9539. If a registration expires, the registrant is no longer authorized to handle controlled substances. Until the registration is renewed and a new certificate of registration is issued, use of the registration is a violation of the law.

4. As noted earlier, DEA registrations are issued for controlled substances activities at a specific location. Federal regulations require that DEA be notified in advance of any change of address. Additionally, the registration address cannot be a post office box. It must be the physical location where the controlled substance activities occur.

5. The Registration Unit can be contacted toll-free at (800) 882-9539. Whenever contacting the DEA regarding an existing registration, provide the DEA registration number.

The DEA's registration program plays an integral role in efforts to prevent the diversion of legitimately produced controlled substances to the illicit market. The program has grown in complexity with the addition of new controlled substances as well as with new automated initiatives. The continued success of the program is the result of the combined efforts and understanding of health care professionals, industry, and the DEA.

The answers to many registration questions and the locations of DEA field offices and registration assistants are listed on the Diversion Control Program Web site, available at *www.DEAdiversion.usdoj.gov*.

National Practitioner Data Bank and Healthcare Integrity and Protection Data Bank

These two federal programs collect specific data nationwide about health care practitioners, providers, and suppliers.

The National Practitioner Data Bank (NPDB) collects and releases information on physicians' medical malpractice payments, adverse licensure actions, adverse clinical privilege actions, adverse professional society membership actions, and exclusions from participation in Medicare and Medicaid. The NPDB is a flagging system that facilitates a comprehensive review of actions affecting health care practitioners' professional credentials. Hospitals, managed care organizations, other authorized health care entities, professional societies, and state licensing boards use NPDB information, in conjunction with other sources, when granting clinical privileges or when making employment, affiliation, or licensure decisions. Hospitals, professional societies, and other health care organizations are also required to report certain data to the NPDB. Malpractice insurers must report all payments made for individual practitioners.

The Healthcare Integrity and Protection Data Bank (HIPDB) collects and releases information on health care practitioners, providers, and suppliers' licensure and certification actions, exclusions from participation in federal and state health care programs, criminal convictions and civil judgments related to health care, and other adjudicated actions or decisions. The HIPDB is an alert or flagging system that assists federal and state agencies, state licensing boards, and health plans in conducting extensive, independent investigations of the qualifications of health care practitioners, providers, or suppliers whom they seek to license, hire, or credential, or with whom they seek to contract or affiliate. Health plans and federal and state government agencies are required to report certain data to the HIPDB.

Both Data Banks are operated under the direct supervision of the Division of Practitioner Data Banks, Bureau of Health Professions, Health Resources and Services Administration, US Department of Health and Human Services (HHS), although the HHS Office of the Inspector General has statutory responsibility for the HIPDB. The NPDB began collecting and disseminating information in 1990. The HIPDB began collecting information in 1999 and disseminating it in 2000.

Data Availability and Confidentiality

Information reported to the NPDB and HIPDB is considered confidential. NPDB information is available only to state licensing boards; hospitals and other health care entities, including professional societies; and others as specified in the law. HIPDB information is available only to health plans and federal and state government agencies. Information that identifies individuals is not available to the general public. Statistical information is made available to the public.

Health care practitioners, providers, and suppliers are allowed to query their own records in the NPDB and HIPDB at any time. All self-query requests are automatically sent to both Data Banks, and a fee of $8 is assessed by each Data Bank. A self-query may not be sent to only one Data Bank. Subjects of a report in either Data Bank receive with their self-query responses a list of all parties to whom the report has been disclosed. To self-query, see: *www.npdb-hipdb.hrsa.gov/welcomesq.html*

Reporting, Statements, and Disputing Reports

NPDB and HIPDB reporting and querying are done electronically through a secure Internet site, at *www.npdb-hipdb.hrsa.gov*. Reporting is combined, with a set of rules determining how reports are accepted into each Data Bank. Based on the information submitted, the NPDB-HIPDB computer system routes reports to the appropriate Data Bank(s). Queriers eligible for both Data Banks may also submit one query that is routed to both.

After processing a report from a reporting entity, the NPDB and HIPDB sends a notice to the entity and to the individual or organizations ("subjects") mentioned in the report. If there are errors, subjects must ask the reporting entity to correct the information. Both Data Banks are prohibited from modifying information submitted in reports except through a "Secretarial Review" process established to resolve disputed reports not corrected by the reporting entities.

Subjects of a NPDB or HIPDB report may add a statement to the report, dispute either the factual accuracy of the information in a report or whether the report was submitted in accordance with NPDB or HIPDB reporting requirements, or both. If the reporting entity does not make a correction satisfactory to the subject of a report, the subject may request "Secretarial Review." The HHS will then review whether the report was legally filed and accurate.

Responsibilities of State Boards

State licensing boards must report to the NPDB certain adverse licensure actions related to professional competence or professional conduct and any changes to such actions. These actions include revocation, suspension, censure, reprimand, probation, and surrender. Boards must also report revisions to adverse licensure actions. State boards must report to the HIPDB final adverse actions taken against health care practitioners, providers, or suppliers.

Available Materials

Materials available from the Data Banks include the *National Practitioner Data Bank Guidebook*; *Healthcare Integrity and Protection Data Bank Guidebook*; fact sheets on various topics; and self-query materials. All of the materials are available on the Internet at *www.npdb-hipdb.hrsa.gov*.

National Practitioner Data Bank and
Healthcare Integrity and Protection Data Bank
PO Box 10832
Chantilly, VA 20153-0832
(800) 767-6732
www.npdb-hipdb.hrsa.gov

Section VI.

Other Organizations and Programs

American Board of Medical Specialties (ABMS)

The American Board of Medical Specialties (ABMS®), a not-for-profit organization, represents 24 approved medical specialty boards that establish and maintain high standards for physician certification and the delivery of safe, quality medical care by certified physician specialists. The primary function of the ABMS is to assist the Member Boards in their efforts to develop and use standards for the evaluation and certification of physician specialists.

Additionally, in collaboration with other organizations and the Accreditation Council for Graduate Medical Education (ACGME), the Member Boards assist in improving the quality of medical education by elevating the standards for graduate medical education and accreditation (approval) of residency and training programs.

The ABMS Member Boards (listed below) have been approved by the ABMS and the AMA Council on Medical Education (AMA CME) through the Liaison Committee for Specialty Boards (LCSB), with ultimate approval of the application by the membership of the ABMS and the AMA CME.

American Board of:

- Allergy and Immunology
- Anesthesiology
- Colon and Rectal Surgery
- Dermatology
- Emergency Medicine
- Family Medicine
- Internal Medicine
- Medical Genetics
- Neurological Surgery
- Nuclear Medicine
- Obstetrics and Gynecology
- Ophthalmology
- Orthopaedic Surgery
- Otolaryngology
- Pathology
- Pediatrics
- Physical Medicine and Rehabilitation
- Plastic Surgery
- Preventive Medicine
- Psychiatry and Neurology
- Radiology
- Surgery
- Thoracic Surgery
- Urology

The governing body of each ABMS Member Board is composed of specialists qualified in the particular field represented by that board. These individuals can include teachers in the specialty, those with specialized training or skills in the primary specialty or subspecialties represented by the Board, and from among those who have demonstrated the expertise, motivation, and ability to assist in the evaluation procedures leading to certification.

About Specialties in Medicine

Specialties in medicine develop because of the rapidly expanding body of knowledge about health and illness and the constantly evolving treatment techniques for disease. Some specialists are primary care doctors, such as family physicians, general internists, and general pediatricians. Other specialists concentrate on certain body systems, specific age groups, or complex scientific techniques developed to diagnose or treat certain types of disorders.

A subspecialist is a physician who has completed training in a general medical/surgical specialty and takes additional training in a more specific area of that specialty called a subspecialty. This training increases the depth of knowledge and expertise of the specialist in that particular field.

Specialty Board Certification and Medical Licensure

To better understand the importance of certification, one must first understand the differences between licensure and certification.

Medical licensure provides a physician with the legal privilege to practice medicine. It is not specialty-specific or designed to recognize the knowledge and skills of a trained specialist, but a legal necessity, granted by state governments, that permits a physician to take on personal and unsupervised responsibility for the diagnosis and treatment of patients in the broad practice of medicine.

Licensure establishes the minimum competence that is essential to protecting the health, safety, and welfare of the public. A physician is granted a license to practice by a state board of medical examiners after completing a certain amount of training and passing a national, and in a few instances a state, licensure examination. Each state or territory has its own procedures to license physicians and sets the general standards for all physicians in that state or territory.

Certification of physician specialists, a practice which has existed for 75 years, is separate from medical licensure and has largely been voluntary. However, with the current forces affecting health care, more and more physicians are being required or are electing to seek formal recognition of their qualifications.

Certification obtained through one of the ABMS Member Boards denotes that a physician has gone beyond the minimum requirement necessary for licensure. It provides the assurance that a physician has the appropriate knowledge, skills, and experience needed to deliver quality care in a specific area of medicine according to the standards designated by the ABMS and its Member Boards.

The ABMS Member Boards oversee the certification process for their particular specialty. A physician receives certification as a specialty medical practitioner after completing an accredited training program, undergoing an evaluation of his or her record by a panel of peer experts, and passing a comprehensive examination given by an ABMS Member Board.

Physicians meeting this set of requirements are awarded general certificates in the field represented by that Member Board. Physicians can also become certified in a subspecialty, a particular area within the specialty, which requires additional training and examination.

Continuous Certification of Physician Specialists

Recognizing that the professional responsibility of physicians requires ongoing learning and improvement throughout their careers, a program of continuous certification called ABMS Maintenance of Certification® (MOC) was developed by the ABMS and the Member Boards as a formal means of measuring a physician's cumulative and ongoing qualifications in the specialty and/or subspecialty in which certification is held.

MOC is a professional development program for physicians who are certified by one of the 24 ABMS Member Boards. The MOC program standards are set by ABMS and independently implemented by the Member Boards. MOC promotes continuous lifelong learning and self assessment to better meet patient, provider, and payer expectations for quality care. It aligns with the movement toward competency-based certification, the increasing evidence that competency degrades over time, the call for enhanced public accountability and credibility, and the potential linkages with periodic maintenance of licensure requirements.

With the MOC program, the ABMS Member Boards are moving away from periodic (every 6, 7, or 10 years) recertification by examination to a more comprehensive process for assessing the continuing competence of physician specialists and their ability to provide quality health care. The MOC processes assure that the physician is maintaining an appropriate level of knowledge in the specialty to promote optimal health outcomes.

The MOC program incorporates the latest research on physician competence, patient safety, and practice management care and focuses on six general competencies:

- Patient care
- Medical knowledge
- Practice-based learning and improvement
- Interpersonal and communications skills
- Professionalism
- Systems-based practice

These areas were identified jointly by the ABMS and the ACGME as those which are crucial for a physician to deliver high-quality patient care.

MOC was initially proposed in 1998-99 and developed with the involvement of a broad spectrum of medical and surgical specialties. The effort is supported by many major medical organizations, including the:

- American Medical Association (AMA)
- American Hospital Association (AHA)
- National Board of Medical Examiners (NBME)
- Federation of State Medical Boards of the US (FSMB)
- The Joint Commission
- Council of Medical Specialty Societies (CMSS)
- Accreditation Council for Graduate Medical Education (ACGME)
- Association of American Medical Colleges (AAMC)
- Educational Commission for Foreign Medical Graduates (ECFMG).

The MOC process has four basic components:

1. Professional standing
Documents that the certified physician has met and maintains legal requirements to practice medicine. All licenses held by a physician must be unrestricted.

2. Lifelong learning and self-assessment
This component enables physicians to reaffirm their commitment to continuous learning and improvement and to assume a leadership role in the quest for safe, quality health care. This requires evidence of participation in educational and self-assessment programs and meeting specialty-specific standards. It is integrated with practice performance to provide a real world practice basis to guide learning and enables physicians to put their learning to use continuously and regularly in the process of normal patient care.

3. Cognitive expertise
Provides evidence, through an examination, that physician specialists have the necessary knowledge to provide quality patient care. Examinations cover the scope and range of the discipline and are clinically relevant.

4. Practice performance assessment
This component focuses on improvement in the quality of care through collaborative efforts with other organizations. Physicians are evaluated in their clinical practice according to specialty-specific standards for patient care. They are provided with feedback and techniques for improvement.

Verifying Physician Certification

For all except those recently certified as specialists by an ABMS Member Board, and not yet entered into the ABMS certification database, and except for a very small number of specialists who do not wish to be listed, the fact of certification may be determined through these public services:

- The "Is Your Doctor Certified?" service on the ABMS Web site (*www.abms.org*)

- The ABMS's toll-free Physician Verification service at 866-ASK-ABMS

- The *Official ABMS Directory of Certified Medical Specialists*® available in most public libraries

These resources are not valid for accrediting done by credentialing organizations or other commercial entities. Groups that perform mass verifications must obtain their information from a recognized source, such as the ABMS, or an ABMS-designated agent. ABMS offers a number of verification services to the medical staff and credentialing professionals and other business users.

For more information about the ABMS, ABMS member boards, the certification of physician specialists, and verifying physician certification, contact:

American Board of Medical Specialties
222 North LaSalle Street, Suite 1500
Chicago, IL 60601
(312) 436-2600
(312) 436-2700 Fax
E-mail: *info@abms.org*
www.abms.org

Accreditation Council for Graduate Medical Education (ACGME)

The Accreditation Council for Graduate Medical Education (ACGME) is a private, nonprofit accrediting organization. Its board of directors comprises individuals elected from slates nominated by five national associations interested in graduate medical education (GME): the American Board of Medical Specialties (ABMS), American Hospital Association (AHA), American Medical Association (AMA), Association of American Medical Colleges (AAMC), and Council of Medical Specialty Societies (CMSS).

The ACGME elects three public directors. The chair of the Council of Review Committee Chairs also serves on the board, along with two voting resident physicians: a resident director nominated by the Resident and Fellow Section of the AMA, with the advice of other national organizations that represent residents, and the chair of the Council of Review Committee Residents. A federal government representative serves as a nonvoting member of the board. Numerous other organizations are invited as observers to the public sessions of the ACGME Board and a number of its Board committees.

Each of the 26 Residency Review Committees (RRCs) sponsored by the ACGME consists of representatives appointed by the AMA, the ABMS specialty board, and, in most cases, the medical specialty society. The Transitional Year Review and Institutional Review Committees are composed of members appointed by the chair of the ACGME in conjunction with the Executive Committee. The term *review committee* is used to denote a Residency Review Committee, Transitional Year Review Committee, or Institutional Review Committee.

GME programs are accredited by the appropriate review committee through authority delegated by the ACGME. Accreditation of a residency program indicates that it is judged to be in substantial compliance with the program requirements for residency education in the particular specialty.

A list of programs accredited by the ACGME, including detailed information about each program, is published annually by the AMA in the *Graduate Medical Education Directory*. The most current listing can be found on the ACGME Web site at *www.acgme.org*.

ACGME General Competencies

In 1999, the ACGME endorsed six General Competencies. ACGME Program Requirements state that GME programs must define the specific knowledge, skills, and attitudes required and provide educational experiences as needed in order for their residents/fellows to demonstrate these competencies to the level expected of a practitioner entering the unsupervised practice of medicine in their chosen discipline.

Patient Care that is compassionate, appropriate, and effective for the treatment of health problems and the promotion of health

Medical Knowledge about established and evolving biomedical, clinical, and cognate (e.g., epidemiological and social-behavioral) sciences and the application of this knowledge to patient care

Practice-Based Learning and Improvement that involves investigation and evaluation of their own patient care, appraisal and assimilation of scientific evidence, and improvements in patient care

Interpersonal and Communication Skills that result in effective information exchange and teaming with patients, their families, and other health professionals

Professionalism, as manifested through a commitment to carrying out professional responsibilities, adherence to ethical principles, and sensitivity to a diverse patient population

Systems-Based Practice, as manifested by actions that demonstrate an awareness of and responsiveness to the larger context and system of health care and the ability to effectively call on system resources to provide care of optimal value

Contact Information

Accreditation Council for Graduate Medical Education
515 N State St, Suite 2000
Chicago, IL 60654
(312) 755-5000
www.acgme.org

Accreditation Council for Continuing Medical Education (ACCME)

The mission of the Accreditation Council for Continuing Medical Education (ACCME) is to identify, develop, and promote standards for quality continuing medical education (CME) utilized by physicians in their maintenance of competence and incorporation of new knowledge to improve quality medical care for patients and their communities.

The ACCME fulfills its mission through a voluntary self-regulated system for accrediting CME providers and a peer-review process responsive to changes in medical education and the health care delivery system.

The primary responsibilities of the ACCME are to:

- Serve as the body accrediting institutions and organizations offering CME

- Serve as the body recognizing institutions and organizations offering CME accreditation

- Develop criteria for evaluation of both educational programs and their activities by which ACCME and state accrediting bodies will accredit institutions and organizations and be responsible for assuring compliance with these standards

- Develop, or foster the development of, methods for measuring the effectiveness of CME and its accreditation, particularly in its relationship to supporting quality patient care and the continuum of medical education

- Recommend and initiate studies for improving the organization and processes of CME and its accreditation

- Review and assess developments in CME's support of quality health

- Review periodically its role in continuing medical education to ensure it remains responsive to public and professional needs.

The ACCME continues to emphasize that CME must be a strategic asset to all stakeholders who seek to improve healthcare in the US. Since 2006, with the announcement of *Updated Accreditation Criteria*, the ACCME has maintained a focus on supporting a well-organized transition to a criterion-based system for the accreditation of CME providers that matches the gaps in physician competence, performance, and patient outcomes (i.e., professional practice gaps) with practice-based learning and change. While putting additional resources into the management of issues to ensure the independence of CME from commercial influence, the ACCME is steadfast in its delivery of a valid accreditation system based upon the 2006 Updated Criteria, which include the ACCME Standards for Commercial Support: Standards to Ensure Independence in CME Activities. SM

The ACCME system includes approximately 730 organizations that are directly accredited by ACCME and another 1,700 organizations accredited within the ACCME's state-based system. The state-based CME system is made up of 46 organizations that are "Recognized" by the ACCME as accreditors of state-based CME providers. Recognition is achieved through ACCME's formal review process. The ACCME's Recognition decision-making is criterion referenced against a predetermined set of standards to ensure equivalency across accreditors. All accreditation decisions made within the ACCME system are based on the 2006 *Updated Accreditation Criteria*.

Contact Information

Accreditation Council for Continuing Medical Education
515 N State St, Suite 1801
Chicago, IL 60654
(312) 527-9200
www.accme.org

American Medical Association Survey and Data Resources

The AMA Division of Survey and Data Resources is dedicated to effectively and accurately collecting, analyzing, and managing physician data within the Physician Masterfile. The AMA Physician Masterfile is a data source not only for AMA internal use but also for use by other professional medical organizations, universities and medical schools, research institutions, governmental agencies, and other related groups. The use of Physician Masterfile data by agencies and organizations concerned with verifying physicians' credentials and health manpower planning is fundamental to the AMA's mission to strengthen the medical profession and ensure quality health care for the American public.

The Physician Masterfile is a database comprising current and historical data for more than 940,000 residents/fellows and physicians and 77,000 students in the United States, both AMA members and nonmembers. This figure includes approximately 243,000 graduates of foreign medical schools who reside in the United States and who have met the educational and credentialing requirements necessary for recognition and approximately 62,000 doctors of osteopathy. Physicians' records are subject to change and are updated continuously through the extensive data collection activities described below.

Survey and Data Resources is composed of the following units:

- Department of Data Integration and Quality Analysis
- Department of Practice and Communication Data
- Information Management and Data Release
- Data Integration and Operation Support

These units are essential in maintaining the Masterfile as one of the most comprehensive and accurate sources of physician data.

Department of Data Integration and Quality Analysis

The responsibility of the Department of Data Integration and Quality Analysis is to ensure that the AMA's Physician Masterfile contains timely and high-quality data on physicians, residents, medical students, medical education institutions, and other healthcare organizations. A core function performed within this department is to establish new AMA Physician Masterfile records, assigning a unique identifier that will remain the same throughout a physician's medical career.

In addition, the department processes resident information collected via the National Graduate Medical Education (GME) Census, an annual survey conducted jointly with the Association of American Medical Colleges (AAMC). Each year, approximately 8,600 ACGME-accredited and 120 ABMS Board-approved GME programs are surveyed. The reported residency information is internally validated and incorporated into a physician's record. The survey also includes questions on GME program characteristics, such as clinical and research facilities and the learning environment, which are used to update FREIDA Online® (*www.ama-assn.org/go/freida*) and the *Graduate Medical Education Directory*, produced by the Division of Graduate Medical Education.

Department of Practice and Communications Data

The responsibility of this department is to track physicians throughout their professional careers by collecting and maintaining current practice and communications data. The Department of Practice and Communications Data surveys up to 375,000 physicians annually, applies updates to more than 300,000 physician mailing addresses per year, and collects updates to group practice locations and physician affiliation data from more than 79,000 US medical groups.

Once physicians complete residency and/or fellowship training, the department tracks them throughout their professional careers. The annual Census of Physicians, for example, is mailed to approximately 250,000 physicians per year and collects information on a physician's professional medical activities, preferred mailing address, principal hospital and group affiliations, and practice specialties, among other data. This department also utilizes over 20 additional sources to supplement data collected via the Physicians Census mailings. The information that is captured is used to support membership efforts, communicate with physicians, segment physician markets, draw samples for health-related research, perform workforce analysis, and track professional trends.

Another primary function of this department is to conduct annual surveys of medical group practices, keeping the Group Practice Database current. This database contains information and affiliations for more than 79,000 group practice locations and 550,000 associated physician affiliations.

Information Management and Data Release

This business unit within the Division of Survey and Data Resources educates others about, facilitates access to, and evaluates the quality of the AMA Physician Masterfile.

The unit educates data users about the Physician Masterfile by managing and responding to telephone, e-mail, and written inquiries regarding Physician Masterfile data, fulfilling more than 300 data requests a year. This effort supports the communications, marketing, and planning efforts of other AMA units.

A primary role of the unit is production of the book *Physician Characteristics and Distribution in the US*, an annual publication with comprehensive statistical data on the physician supply in the United States. In addition, Data Release Services supports the AMA's Partnership for Growth Data Reciprocity Project, which promotes data sharing with state medical associations and national medical specialty organizations.

Data Integration and Operation Support

Within the division office, this business unit is responsible for processing over 40 million updates annually received from state regulatory and federal agencies, medical specialty groups and organizations, educational and training institutions, and membership and subscription services. Of utmost importance to the division is ensuring timely data load cycles to the Masterfile. On average, 97% of the matched records are loaded to the Masterfile within six business days of receipt. Timely processing of incoming data is key to ensuring accurate and comprehensive reporting to credentialing groups and health care organizations.

Other activities performed within the division include:

- Managing the AMA's corporate mailing list application, which includes more than 100 different list directories and supports key Association activities involving the AMA board, councils, committees, advisory groups, and House of Delegates

- Publishing the Federation and Pictorial Directories on the AMA Web site

- Providing a mechanism and data resources for use by medical schools, universities, research institutions, governmental agencies, and other organizations interested in the study of heath care policy issues

- Coordinating the distribution of Masterfile-related reports, physician profiles, and data to state, county, and national specialty medical societies

- Conducting validation studies

- Developing, measuring, and monitoring key performance indicators

- Identifying, researching, and analyzing potential new sources of data as well as new tools to enhance data processing.

Contact Information

Division of Survey and Data Resources
Monica Quiroz, Director
monica.quiroz@ama-assn.org

Data Integration and Quality Analysis
Mark Long, Director
mark.long@ama-assn.org

Department of Practice and Communications Data
Susan Montrimas, Director
susan.montrimas@ama-assn.org

Information Management and Data Release
Derek Smart, Manager
derek.smart@ama-assn.org

American Medical Association Continuing Medical Education

Advances in biomedical science and changes in the other facets of the US health care delivery environment engage physicians in a continuous process of professional development. To ensure that they provide patients with the most current and appropriate treatment, services, and information, physicians continue learning through participation in a wide array of structured educational activities, as well as through independent study. The American Medical Association (AMA) supports these physician efforts by:

- Administering the only non-specialty-specific credit system that recognizes physician completion of continuing medical education (CME) activities—the AMA PRA credit system

- Establishing learning modalities (e.g., performance improvement CME [PI CME] and Internet point of care [PoC]) to enhance physician professional development and improve patient care

- Establishing agreements to enable US physicians to obtain *AMA PRA Category 1 Credit*™ for participation in international meetings

- Offering certified CME activities (live, journal-based manuscript review, enduring materials, and performance improvement CME)

The AMA Physician's Recognition Award

In 1968, the AMA House of Delegates established the AMA Physician's Recognition Award (PRA) to both encourage physicians to participate in CME and acknowledge when individual physicians complete CME activities. Activities that meet education standards established by the AMA can be designated for *AMA PRA Category 1 Credit*™ by educational institutions accredited to provide CME to physicians through the Accreditation Council for Continuing Medical Education (ACCME) or an ACCME-recognized state medical society. These accredited CME providers typically include state medical societies, medical specialty societies, medical schools, and hospitals. Other activities, usually independent or physician directed learning, may be reported for *AMA PRA Category 2 Credit*™.

AMA PRA certificates are awarded in lengths of 1, 2, or 3 years, with the following requirements:

1-year certificate – 50 credits
- 20 AMA PRA Category 1 Credits
- 30 AMA PRA Category 1 or AMA PRA Category 2 Credits

2-year certificate – 100 credits
- 40 AMA PRA Category 1 Credits
- 60 AMA PRA Category 1 or AMA PRA Category 2 Credits

3-year certificate – 150 credits
- 60 AMA PRA Category 1 Credits
- 90 AMA PRA Category 1 or AMA PRA Category 2 Credits

The AMA also offers the AMA PRA with Commendation, awarded to physicians who exceed the credits required to earn the standard AMA PRA. For more information, visit *www.ama-assn.org/go/pra*.

Through reciprocity arrangements, the AMA will also award the AMA PRA certificate if the CME requirements of the following organizations are met:

- American Academy of Dermatology
- American Academy of Family Physicians
- American Academy of Ophthalmology
- American Academy of Pediatrics
- American College of Obstetricians and Gynecologists
- American Psychiatric Association
- American Society of Plastic Surgeons
- American Urological Association Education and Research, Inc
- California Medical Association
- Medical Society of New Jersey
- Pennsylvania Medical Society

Many state and territory licensing jurisdictions will accept the PRA certificate or approved application as evidence that physicians have met the CME requirements for licensure. A list of these states can be found in Table 16, Continuing Medical Education for Licensure Reregistration.

The Joint Commission will accept, subject to review, correctly completed AMA PRA applications stamped "approved" by the AMA as documented physician compliance with The Joint Commission's CME requirements.

The AMA sends reminders to physicians whose current certificate is expiring within the next 6 months. The AMA PRA application form and the PRA Information Booklet, respectively, are available online at

www.ama-assn.org/go/applypra
www.ama-assn.org/go/prabooklet

Department of AMA PRA Standards and Policy
Continuing Physician Professional Development
American Medical Association
515 N State St
Chicago, IL 60654
(312) 464-4941
(312) 464-4567 Fax
E-mail: pra@ama-assn.org

AMA-accredited CME Programs

Conferences and Live Events

As an ACCME-accredited provider, the AMA sponsors multiple conferences and live events designated for AMA PRA Category 1 Credit. Physicians may participate in education on topics of interest to all disciplines and specialties. Recent AMA-sponsored or cosponsored conferences and live events include Basic and Advanced Disaster Life Support programs, Assessing and Counseling Older Drivers workshops, and Group and Faculty Practice Web Conferences.

AMA Enduring Materials

The AMA offers a number of enduring CME activities for physicians. These modules offer quality CME in a convenient format that permits learners to work at their own pace and at a time that fits a busy clinical schedule. Available in print, CD-ROM, and Internet formats, these enduring CME activities are dedicated to improving the effectiveness and scope of CME by using new formats and delivery approaches and incorporating the latest clinical information. An updated list of available programs can be accessed at www.ama-assn.org/go/cme.

Journal CME

The AMA has launched online journal CME activities in the *Journal of the American Medical Association (JAMA)* and in the following six AMA *Archives* journals.

- *Archives of Dermatology*
- *Archives of Internal Medicine*
- *Archives of Neurology*
- *Archives of Ophthalmology*
- *Archives of Otolaryngology—Head and Neck Surgery*
- *Archives of Surgery*

Physicians can earn AMA PRA Category 1 Credit by reading the designated articles online and completing a post-test.

Other Activities

The AMA also provides opportunities for physicians to earn *AMA PRA Category 1 Credit*™ through participation in manuscript review for *JAMA* and the *Archives* and select PI CME activities.

International CME

The International Conference Recognition (ICR) Program began in 1990 by an act of the AMA House of Delegates. The AMA recognized that international congresses present opportunities for physicians to participate in quality educational programs and provide opportunities for US physicians to collaborate with colleagues in other countries.

The AMA recognizes several events each year and provides American physicians with an opportunity to earn AMA PRA Category 1 Credit at these approved events. For more information, visit *www.ama-assn.org/go/internationalcme*.

The AMA also has an agreement with the European Union of Medical Specialties to convert European Accreditation Council for Continuing Medical Education (EACCME) credit to AMA PRA Category 1 Credit for physicians that attend international conferences that are designated for EACCME credit. For more information, see: *www.ama-assn.org/go/internationalcme*

Contact Information

For more information on AMA CME programs and activities, visit *www.ama-assn.org/go/cme* or contact:

AMA CME activities	(312) 464-4637
AMA CME credits	(312) 464-4941
Physician's Recognition Award	(312) 464-4941
International Recognition Program	(312) 464-5196
EACCME credit conversion	(312) 464-5296
AMA PRA Credit System	(312) 464-4668

For general information, contact:

Continuing Physician Professional Development
American Medical Association
515 N State St
Chicago, IL 60654
(312) 464-4671
(312) 464-5830 Fax
E-mail: *cppd@ama-assn.org*

The Joint Commission

An independent, nonprofit organization, The Joint Commission evaluates and accredits more than 16,000 health care organizations and programs in the United States. Accreditation by The Joint Commission is recognized nationwide as a symbol of quality that reflects an organization's commitment to meeting certain performance standards.

The Joint Commission develops its standards in consultation with health care experts, practitioners, providers, measurement experts, purchasers, and consumers. The standards focus on an organization's ability to provide safe, high-quality care and on its actual performance.

To earn and maintain accreditation, an organization must undergo an unannounced on-site survey by a team of Joint Commission surveyors at least every 3 years (laboratories are surveyed every 2 years). The Joint Commission employs experienced physicians, nurses, health care administrators, medical technologists, psychologists, pharmacists, and other medical professionals to conduct these surveys.

Accreditation Programs

The Joint Commission operates the following accreditation programs, which serve various types of health care organizations:

- Hospital Accreditation Program
- Home Care Accreditation Program
- Ambulatory Care Accreditation Program
- Laboratory Accreditation Program
- Long-Term Care Accreditation Program
- Behavioral Health Care Accreditation Program
- Critical Access Hospital Accreditation Program
- Office-Based Surgery Accreditation Program

International accreditation services are provided through Joint Commission International, a subsidiary of The Joint Commission.

The Joint Commission also awards Disease-Specific Care Certification, designed to evaluate clinical programs for virtually any chronic disease or condition. The Joint Commission's Health Care Staffing Services Certification program evaluates a staffing firm's ability to provide qualified and competent staffing services.

Benefits of Accreditation and Certification

Accreditation and certification by The Joint Commission offers the following benefits:

- Strengthens community confidence in the quality and safety of care, treatment, and services

- Provides a competitive edge in the marketplace

- Improves risk management and risk reduction

- Provides education on good practices to improve business operations

- Provides professional advice and counsel, enhancing staff education

- Enhances staff recruitment and development

- Is recognized by select insurers and other third parties

- May fulfill regulatory requirements in select states

Major Initiatives

The Joint Commission works to improve the safety and quality of health care through its Sentinel Event Database and the ORYX initiative. The database permits dissemination of lessons learned from analysis of serious adverse events by accredited organizations and serves as a basis for the annual issuance of National Patient Safety Goals. ORYX measurements supplement and help guide the standards-based survey process by providing a more targeted basis for the regular accreditation survey, for continuously monitoring actual performance, and for guiding and stimulating continuous improvement in health care organizations.

The Joint Commission convenes an ongoing series of Public Policy Roundtables. Each Roundtable culminates in a national summit and the publication of a white paper with explicit recommendations and assigned accountabilities. White papers on the nurse staffing crisis, emergency preparedness, organ donation, health literacy, and tort resolution and patient safety have received extensive national attention. Roundtables have also addressed emergency department overcrowding, health professions education reform, the hospital of the future, waste reduction, and creation of a national data management strategy.

In March 2002, The Joint Commission, together with the Centers for Medicare and Medicaid Services, launched a national campaign known as Speak Up™ to urge patients to take a role in preventing health care errors by becoming active, involved, and informed participants on the health care team. Speak Up™ campaigns have included:

- Help prevent errors in your care
- Help avoid mistakes in your surgery
- Information for living organ donors
- Five things you can do to prevent infection
- Help avoid mistakes with your medicines
- What you should know about research studies
- Planning your follow-up care
- Help prevent medical test mistakes
- Know your rights
- Understanding your doctors and other caregivers

Consumers can find information about Joint Commission-accredited and -certified health care organizations online through Quality Check™, which is accessible at *www.qualitycheck.org*. Quality reports that provide detailed performance information about each accredited organization are also available through Quality Check. The Joint Commission issues an annual report that contains aggregate data on the quality and safety-related performance of America's hospitals.

Origins/Governance

The Joint Commission was founded in 1951. Its governing Board of Commissioners consists of 29 individuals whose backgrounds and experience reflect a broad range of professional and lay interests. The board includes practicing physicians, nurses, administrators, quality experts, ethicists, and educators, as well as a labor representative and a consumer advocate. The Board of Commissioners brings to The Joint Commission diverse experience in health care, business, and public policy.

Contact Information

The Joint Commission
One Renaissance Blvd
Oakbrook Terrace, IL 60181
(630) 792-5000
(630) 792-5005 Fax
www.jointcommission.org

National Committee for Quality Assurance (NCQA)

The National Committee for Quality Assurance (NCQA) is a private, not-for-profit organization that assesses and reports on the quality of health care services in multiple areas of the health care system to provide a basis for quality improvement activities and for public reporting of performance. The efforts of NCQA are organized around programs providing accreditation and certification of organizations, including health plans and other entities, and recognition programs for individual clinical practices.

Origins and Scope

The NCQA began evaluating and accrediting managed care organizations in 1991 in response to the need for standardized, objective information about the quality of these organizations. Since then, it has expanded the range of organizations that it accredits or certifies to include human subject research protection programs, managed behavioral health care organizations, credentials verification organizations, physician organizations, and others. NCQA has also developed, in collaboration with organizations such as the American Diabetes Association and American Heart Association/American Stroke Association, recognition programs that evaluate and report on the quality of care at the individual physician level.

MCO Accreditation

The NCQA accreditation process is best illustrated by its MCO (managed care organization) accreditation program. More than 75% of individuals enrolled in HMOs are in plans currently accredited by NCQA. Organizations seeking NCQA accreditation must report via a Web-based tool (the Interactive Survey System) their adherence to standards that evaluate the health plan's clinical and administrative systems, including efforts to continuously improve the quality of care and service it delivers. In addition, plans are required to report, and are scored on their performance on, a set of clinical quality measures (Health Plan Employer Data and Information Set, or HEDIS®; see next page).

Plans are reviewed against and scored on more than 50 standards and on clinical measures in the following categories:

- Quality improvement
- Credentialing
- Members' rights and responsibilities
- Preventive health services
- Utilization management
- Medical records
- Performance on HEDIS measures (clinical and patient experiences)

NCQA accreditation surveys are conducted by teams of physicians and managed care experts. A national oversight committee of physicians analyzes the team's findings and assigns one of five possible accreditation levels (excellent, commendable, accredited, provisional, or denied) based on the plan's level of compliance with NCQA standards. NCQA's MCO accreditation process is thus unique among accreditation programs in its use of direct measures of clinical performance in scoring of accreditation. A significant new, and currently voluntary, module within the health plan accreditation program, Physician Hospital Quality (PHQ), sets standards for plans related to their evaluation of physician and hospital quality.

Recognition Programs

In response to the demand for evaluation of ambulatory care quality, NCQA developed, in partnership with the ADA, a Diabetes Physician Recognition Program® (DPRP) and with the AHA/ASA the Heart-Stroke Recognition Program® (HSRP), as well as the recently developed Back Pain Recognition Program® (BPRP). It has also developed a recognition program (the Physician Practice Connections® program or PPC) that examines the degree to which an office practice has incorporated systems (such as registries, care management, etc) into the practice. This program has been adapted and endorsed for use in qualifying practices in patient-centered medical home (PCMH) demonstration and pilot projects by the American College of Physicians, American Academy of Family Physicians, American

Academy of Pediatrics, and American Osteopathic Association, and a slightly modified version, known as PPC_PCMH-CMS, will be used in the CMS PCMH demonstration project. Thresholds for achieving recognition in each of the programs are set by expert panels of clinicians and others. Practices that wish to receive recognition submit data and documentation to NCQA, which evaluates the data against the predetermined threshold values. The NCQA recognition programs have been adopted by a number of pay-for-performance initiatives, including the GE-led Bridges to Excellence® program. A variety of other recognition programs are currently in development.

Performance Measurement

HEDIS® and related NCQA Clinical Measures

NCQA manages the most widely used set of performance measurements for evaluating quality in ambulatory care, HEDIS®. This measurement set, which includes more than 75 fully specified and standardized measures, is used to evaluate health care quality aggregated at the health plans level. NCQA has also created a companion set of measures for use in reporting at the physician office practice level, including those used in the various physician recognition programs. Nearly all of the physician-level measures have been endorsed by the National Quality Forum (NQF). NCQA has also worked with the AMA-sponsored Physician Consortium on Performance Improvement on developing a broad set of clinical measures for the CMS-sponsored Physician Quality Reporting Incentive program (PQRI)

Work related to measurement has led NCQA to develop projects and programs related to distribution and reporting of performance data, ensuring data accuracy, and making sure the performance data are useful to help guide choice.

In summary, NCQA's work in the area of health care evaluation focuses on four key areas: accreditation, recognition programs, data audit oversight, and collection of HEDIS® and related measures. NCQA publicly reports performance data through Quality Compass® (a national database of HEDIS® data and accreditation information) as well as various other evaluation reports for physicians, plans, consumers, and purchasers.

Contact Information

National Committee for Quality Assurance
1100 13th St, NW
Washington, DC 20056
(202) 955-3500
(202) 955-3599 Fax
www.ncqa.org

Administrators in Medicine (AIM)

Administrators in Medicine (AIM), a not-for-profit organization, is the national organization for state medical and osteopathic board executives. Founded in 1984, AIM has the mission of assisting and supporting administrators for medical licensing and regulatory authorities to achieve administrative excellence and ultimately advance public safety. AIM offers educational, research, and online services for its membership, both in the US and, increasingly, internationally. AIM's public outreach is via the online search engine it provides along with board Web links on its nationally recognized *AIM DocFinder* Web site.

Education is the cornerstone of what AIM does as an organization for member board executives. AIM sponsors a variety of educational seminars, including AIM Regional Meetings, where board executives discuss operational issues. Its AIM Institute Educational Workshops—Physician Licensing, Profiles and Technology—provide an excellent overview of best practices and how to avoid pitfalls and are presented by an expert faculty of board senior staff and experts from the credentialing and technology fields. Its Annual Meeting educational program provides an opportunity to hear from national experts in a variety of fields impacting medical licensure and discipline.

AIM's *State Medical Board Investigator Certification Program* seeks to address the need for highly trained medical board investigators. AIM will create a specialized, focused training program that will provide education and resources for individuals conducting investigations for state medical and osteopathic boards. It will be a well-rounded program that includes basic investigation techniques as well as exposure to the entire system of medical licensure and discipline.

The AIM DocFinder

The AIM *DocFinder* was the only online physician directory of its kind when it was established in 1996. *DocFinder* contains the licensing background and disciplinary information of physicians and other health care practitioners, in addition to physician profile information from states that have passed physician profile laws. Popular with consumers, *DocFinder* is still recognized for its easy-to-use search engine. It has been featured in numerous state and national publications such as *Newsweek* and *The Wall Street Journal* as well as national and local news broadcasts. It remains the only combined database of all licensing jurisdictions that has its direct source of data from and is controlled by state licensing boards and remains free of charge to the public. Access the AIM *DocFinder* at www.docboard.org.

Appendixes

Appendix A

Boards of Medical Examiners in the United States and Possessions

Updated August 2009

Alabama State Board of Medical Examiners
848 Washington Ave
PO Box 946
Montgomery, AL 36101-0946
(334) 242-4116
(334) 242-4155 Fax
www.albme.org

Alaska State Medical Board
550 W Seventh Ave, Ste 1500
Anchorage, AK 99501
(907) 269-8163
(907) 269-8196 Fax
www.commerce.state.ak.us/occ/pmed.htm

Arizona Medical Board
9545 E Doubletree Ranch Rd
Scottsdale, AZ 85258-5514
(480) 551-2700
(480) 551-2704 Fax
www.azmd.gov

Arkansas State Medical Board
2100 Riverfront Dr
Little Rock, AR 72202-1793
(501) 296-1802
(501) 603-3555
www.armedicalboard.org

Medical Board of California
2005 Evergreen St, Ste 1200
Sacramento, CA 95815
(916) 263-2389
(916) 263-2387 Fax
www.medbd.ca.gov

Colorado Board of Medical Examiners
1560 Broadway, Ste 1300
Denver, CO 80202-5140
(303) 894-7690
(303) 894-7692 Fax
www.dora.state.co.us/medical

Connecticut Medical Examining Board
Physician Licensure Unit
PO Box 340308, 410 Capital Ave, MS 13PHO
Hartford, CT 06134-0308
(860) 509-7648
(860) 509-7553 Fax
www.dph.state.ct.us

Delaware Board of Medical Examiners
861 Silver Lake Blvd, Ste 203
Cannon Building
Dover, DE 19904
(302) 744-4500
(302) 739-2711 Fax
www.dpr.delaware.gov

District of Columbia Board of Medicine
Health Professional Licensing Administration
717 14th St NW, Rm 1007
Washington, DC 20005
(202) 724-8800
(202) 727-8471 Fax
www.dchealth.dc.gov

Florida Board of Medicine
Bin #C03
4052 Bald Cypress Way
Tallahassee, FL 32399-3253
(850) 245-4131
(850) 488-9325 Fax
www.doh.state.fl.us

Georgia Composite State Board of Medical Examiners
2 Peachtree St NW, 36th Floor
Atlanta, GA 30303
(404) 656-3913
(404) 656-9723 Fax
www.medicalboard.state.ga.us

Guam Board of Medical Examiners
651 Legacy Square Commercial Complex
S Route 10, Ste 9
Marfilao, GU 96913
(671) 735-7406
(671) 735-7413 Fax

Hawaii Board of Medical Examiners
335 Merchant St, Rm 301
PO Box 3469
Honolulu, HI 96813
(808) 586-2689
(808) 586-2874 Fax
www.ehawaii.gov

Idaho State Board of Medicine
1755 Westgate Dr, Ste 140
Boise, ID 83704
(208) 327-7000
(208) 327-7005 Fax
www.bom.state.id.us

Illinois Medical Licensing Board
Department of Professional Regulation
320 W Washington, 3rd Floor
Springfield, IL 62786
(217) 557-3209
(217) 524-2169
www.idfpr.com

Medical Licensing Board of Indiana
402 W Washington St, Rm W072
Indianapolis, IN 46204
(317) 234-2060
(317) 233-4236 Fax
www.in.gov/pla/medical.htm

Iowa Board of Medicine
400 SW 8th St, Ste C
Des Moines, IA 50309-4686
(515) 281-6641
(515) 242-5908 Fax
www.medicalboard.iowa.gov

Kansas Board of Healing Arts
235 S Topeka Blvd
Topeka, KS 66603-3068
(785) 296-8561
(785) 296-0852 Fax
www.ksbha.org

Kentucky Board of Medical Licensure
Hurstbourne Office Park
310 Whittington Pkwy, Ste 1B
Louisville, KY 40222-4916
(502) 429-7150
(502) 429-7158 Fax
http://kbml.ky.gov

Louisiana State Board of Medical Examiners
630 Camp St
PO Box 30250
New Orleans, LA 70190-0250
(504) 568-6820 x262
(504) 568-8893 Fax
www.lsbme.la.gov

Maine Board of Licensure in Medicine
161 Capitol St
137 State House Station
Augusta, ME 04333
(207) 287-3601
(207) 287-6590 Fax
www.docboard.org/me/me_home.htm

Maryland Board of Physicians
PO Box 2571
4201 Patterson Ave, 4th Floor
Baltimore, MD 21215-0095
(410) 764-4777
(410) 358-2252 Fax
www.mbp.state.md.us

Massachusetts Board of Registration in Medicine
560 Harrison Ave, Ste G-4
Boston, MA 02118
(617) 654-9800
(617) 451-9568 Fax
www.massmedboard.org

Michigan Board of Medicine
611 W Ottawa St, 1st Floor
PO Box 30670
Lansing, MI 48933
(517) 373-6873
(517) 373-2179
www.michigan.gov/healthlicense

Minnesota Board of Medical Practice
University Park Plaza
2829 University Ave SE, Ste 400
Minneapolis, MN 55414-3246
(612) 617-2130
(612) 617-2166 Fax
www.bmp.state.mn.us

Mississippi State Board of Medical Licensure
1867 Crane Ridge Dr, Ste 200B
Jackson, MS 39216
(601) 987-3079
(601) 987-4159 Fax
www.msbml.state.ms.us

Missouri State Board of Registration for the Healing Arts
Division of Professional Registration
3605 Missouri Blvd
Jefferson City, MO 65109
(573) 751-0098
(573) 751-3166 Fax
www.pr.mo.gov/healingarts.asp

Montana Board of Medical Examiners
PO Box 200513
301 S Park Ave, 4th Floor
Helena, MT 59620-0513
(406) 841-2364
(406) 841-2305 Fax
www.medicalboard.mt.gov

Nebraska Board of Medicine and Surgery
Regulation and Licensure Credentialing Division
301 Centennial Mall South, PO Box 94986
Lincoln, NE 68509-4986
(402) 471-2118
(402) 471-3577 Fax
www.hhs.state.ne.us

Nevada State Board of Medical Examiners
1105 Terminal Way, Ste 301
Reno, NV 89502
(775) 688-2559
(775) 688-2321 Fax
www.medboard.nv.gov

New Hampshire Board of Medicine
2 Industrial Park Dr, Ste 8
Concord, NH 03301-8520
(603) 271-1205
(603) 271-6702 Fax
www.state.nh.us/medicine

New Jersey State Board of Medical Examiners
PO Box 183
140 E Front St, 2nd Floor
Trenton, NJ 08625-0183
(609) 826-7100
(609) 826-7117 Fax
www.state.nj.us/lps/ca/medical.htm

New Mexico Medical Board
2055 S Pacheco St
Building 400
Santa Fe, NM 87505
(505) 476-7220
(505) 476-7233 Fax
www.nmmb.state.nm.us/

New York State Board of Medicine
89 Washington Ave
Room 306
Albany, NY 12234
(518) 474-3817 x560
(518) 486-4846 Fax
www.op.nysed.gov

North Carolina Medical Board
1203 Front St
PO Box 20007
Raleigh, NC 27619
(919) 326-1100 ext 218
(919) 326-1131 Fax
www.ncmedboard.org

North Dakota State Board of Medical Examiners
418 E Broadway Ave, Ste 12
Bismarck, ND 58501
(701) 328-6500
(701) 328-6505 Fax
www.ndbomex.com

State Medical Board of Ohio
30 E Broad St, 3rd Floor
Columbus, OH 43215-6127
(614) 466-3934
(614) 728-5946 Fax
www.med.ohio.gov

Oklahoma State Board of Medical Licensure and Supervision
PO Box 18256
Oklahoma City, OK 73154-0256
(405) 848-6841
(405) 848-4999 Fax
www.okmedicalboard.org

Oregon Board of Medical Examiners
1500 SW First Ave
620 Crown Plaza
Portland, OR 97201-5826
(503) 229-5770
(503) 229-6543 Fax
www.bme.state.or.us

Pennsylvania State Board of Medicine
2601 North Third St
PO Box 2649
Harrisburg, PA 17105-2649
(717) 783-1400
(717) 787-7769 Fax
www.dos.state.pa.us

Board of Medical Examiners of Puerto Rico
PO Box 13969
San Juan, PR 00908
(787) 782-8949 or 782-8937
(787) 792-4436 Fax

Rhode Island Board of Medical Licensure and Discipline
Cannon Bldg, Rm 205
Three Capitol Hill
Providence, RI 02908-5097
(401) 222-3855
(401) 222-2158 Fax
www.health.ri.gov/hsr/bmld

South Carolina Board of Medical Examiners
Department of Labor, Licensing & Regulation
110 Centerview Dr, Ste 202
Columbia, SC 29210-1289
(803) 896-4500
(803) 896-4515 Fax
www.llr.state.sc.us/pol/medical

South Dakota State Board of Medical and Osteopathic Examiners
101 N Main Ave, Ste 301
Sioux Falls, SD 57104
(605) 367-7781
(605) 367-7786 Fax
http://medicine.sd.gov

Tennessee Board of Medical Examiners
227 French Landing #300
Nashville, TN 37243
(615) 532-3202
(615) 253-4484 Fax
www.state.tn.us/health

Texas Medical Board
PO Box 2018
Austin, TX 78768-2018
(512) 305-7010
(512) 305-7008 Fax
www.tmb.state.tx.us

Utah Department of Commerce
Division of Occupational & Professional Licensure
PO Box 146741
Salt Lake City, UT 84114-6741
(801) 530-6621
(801) 530-6511 Fax
www.dopl.utah.gov

Vermont Board of Medical Practice
108 Cherry St
PO Box 70
Burlington, VT 05402-0070
(802) 657-4220
(802) 657-4227 Fax
http://healthvermont.gov/hc/med_board/bmp.aspx

Virginia Board of Medicine
9960 Mayland Dr, Ste 300
Richmond, VA 23233-1463
(804) 367-4600
(804) 527-4426 Fax
www.dhp.virginia.gov

Virgin Islands Board of Medical Examiners
Office of the Commissioner, Department of Health
48 Sugar Estate
St Thomas, VI 00802
(340) 774-0117
(340) 777-4001 Fax

Washington Medical Quality Assurance Commision
Department of Health
PO Box 47866
Olympia, WA 98504-7866
(360) 236-4790
(360) 236-4573 Fax
www.doh.wa.gov

West Virginia Board of Medicine
101 Dee Dr
Charleston, WV 25311
(304) 558-2921 x 227
(304) 558-2084 Fax
www.wvdhhr.org/wvbom

State of Wisconsin Medical Examining Board
Dept of Regulation & Licensing
PO Box 8935
Madison, WI 53703-8935
(608) 266-2112
(608) 267-3816 Fax
http://drl.wi.gov

Wyoming Board of Medicine
320 W 25th St, Ste 103
Cheyenne, WY 82002
(307) 778-7053
(307) 778-2069
http://wyomedboard.state.wy.us

Appendix B

Boards of Osteopathic Medical Examiners in the United States and Possessions

Updated August 2009

Arizona Board of Osteopathic Medical Examiners
9535 E Doubletree Ranch Rd
Scottsdale, AZ 85258-5539
(480) 657-7703 x22
(480) 657-7715 Fax
www.azdo.gov

Osteopathic Medical Board of California
1300 National Drive, #150
Sacramento, CA 95834
(916) 928-8390
(916) 928-8392 Fax
www.ombc.ca.gov

Florida Board of Osteopathic Medicine
Bin #C06
4052 Bald Cypress Way
Tallahassee, FL 32399-1753
(850) 245-4161
(850) 487-9874 Fax
www.doh.state.fl.us/mqa

Maine Board of Osteopathic Licensure
142 State House Station
Augusta, ME 04333-0142
(207) 287-2480
(207) 287-3015 Fax
www.maine.gov/osteo

Michigan Board of Osteopathic Medicine and Surgery
611 W Ottawa St, 1st Floor
Lansing, MI 48933
(517) 373-6873
(517) 373-2179 Fax
www.michigan.gov/healthlicense

Nevada State Board of Osteopathic Medicine
2860 E Flamingo Rd, Ste D
Las Vegas, NV 89121
(702) 732-2147
(702) 732-2079 Fax
www.osteo.state.nv.us

New Mexico Board of Osteopathic Medical Examiners
2550 Cerrillos Road
Santa Fe, NM 87505
(505) 476-4695
(505) 476-7095 Fax
www.rld.state.nm.us/osteopathy

Oklahoma Board of Osteopathic Examiners
4848 N Lincoln Blvd, Ste 100
Oklahoma City, OK 73105-3321
(405) 528-8625
(405) 557-0653 Fax
www.ok.gov/osboe/

Pennsylvania State Board of Osteopathic Medicine
PO Box 2649
Harrisburg, PA 17101
(717) 783-4858
(717) 787-7769 Fax
www.dos.state.pa.us

Tennessee State Board of Osteopathic Examiners
First Floor Cordell Hull Bldg
425 5th Ave North
Nashville, TN 37247-1010
(615) 741-4540
(615) 253-4484 Fax
www.state.tn.us/health

State of Utah Department of Commerce
Division of Occupational & Professional Licensing
PO Box 146741
Salt Lake City, UT 84114-6741
(801) 530-6621
(801) 530-6511 Fax
www.dopl.utah.gov

Vermont Board of Osteopathic Physicians and Surgeons
Office of Professional Regulation
National Life Building, North Floor 2
Montpelier, VT 05620-3402
(802) 828-2367
(802) 828-2465
www.sec.state.vt.us

Washington Board of Osteopathic Medicine and Surgery
Department of Health
PO Box 47852
Olympia, WA 98504-7852
(360) 236-4943
(360) 236-2406 Fax
www.doh.wa.gov

West Virginia Board of Osteopathy
334 Penco Rd
Weirton, WV 26062
(304) 723-4638
(304) 723-2877 Fax
www.wvbdosteo.org

Appendix C

Member Organizations of the Federation of Medical Regulatory Authorities of Canada

Updated June 10, 2009

Fleur-Ange Lefebvre, Executive Director and CEO
Federation of Medical Regulatory Authorities of Canada
103 - 2283 St Laurent Blvd, Ste 103
Ottawa, ON K1G 5A2
(613) 738-0372
www.fmrac.ca

Trevor Theman, MD, Registrar
College of Physicians and Surgeons of Alberta
2700 Telus Plaza South
10020 - 100 Street NW
Edmonton, AB T5J 0N3
(780) 423-4764
www.cpsa.ab.ca

Heidi Oetter, MD, Registrar
College of Physicians and Surgeons of British Columbia
400-858 Beatty St
Vancouver, BC V6B 1C1
(604) 733-7758
www.cpsbc.ca

William Pope, MD, Registrar
College of Physicians and Surgeons of Manitoba
1000-1661 Portage Ave
Winnipeg, MB R3J 3T7
(204) 774-4344
www.cpsm.mb.ca

Edmund Schollenberg, MD, Registrar
College of Physicians and Surgeons of New Brunswick
One Hampton Rd, Ste 300
Rothesay, NB E2E 5K8
(506) 849-5050
www.cpsnb.org

Robert W. Young, MD, Registrar
College of Physicians and Surgeons of Newfoundland and Labrador
139 Water St, Ste 603
St John's, NL A1C 1B2
(709) 726-8546
www.cpsnl.ca

Cameron Little, MD, Registrar
College of Physicians and Surgeons of Nova Scotia
200-1559 Brunswick St, Sentry Place
Halifax, NS B3J 2G1
(902) 422-5823
www.cpsns.ns.ca

Barbara Harvey, Registrar, Professional Services
Department of Health Social Services
Government of Nunavut
Box 390
Kugluktuk, NU X0B 0E0
(867) 982-7668
E-mail: *bvandenassem@gov.nu.ca*

Jeannette Hall, Registrar
Department of Health Social Service
Government of the Northwest Territories
Centre Square Tower, 8th Fl, PO Box 1320
Yellowknife, NT X1A 2L9
(867) 920-8058
E-mail: *jeannette_hall@gov.nt.ca*

Rocco Gerace, MD, Registrar
College of Physicians and Surgeons of Ontario
80 College St
Toronto, ON M5G 2E2
(416) 967-2600
www.cpso.on.ca

Cyril Moyse, MD, Registrar
College of Physicians and Surgeons of Prince Edward Island
199 Grafton St
Charlottetown, PE C1A 1L2
(902) 566-3861
www.cpspei.ca

Yves Robert, MD, Secrétaire-général
College des médecins du Québec
2170 boul René Lévésque ouest
Montréal, QC H3H 2T8
(514) 933-4441
www.cmq.org

Dennis A. Kendel, MD, Registrar
College of Physicians and Surgeons of Saskatchewan
500-321A 21st East
Saskatoon, SK S7K 0C1
(306) 244-7355
www.quadrant.net/cpss

Fiona Charbonneau, Registrar
Yukon Medical Council
PO Box 2703 (c-18)
Whitehorse, Yukon Y1A 2C6
(867) 667-3774
www.yukonmedicalcouncil.ca

Appendix D

Glossary of Medical Licensure Terms

Accreditation Council for Graduate Medical Education (ACGME)

Note: See page 129 for more information.

An accrediting agency with the mission of improving health care by assessing and advancing the quality of resident physicians' education through accreditation. The ACGME establishes national standards for graduate medical education by which it approves and continually assesses educational programs under its aegis. The ACGME accredits GME programs through its 28 review committees (26 Residency Review Committees, or RRCs, the Transitional Year Review Committee, and the Institutional Review Committee). The ACGME has five member organizations:

- American Board of Medical Specialties
- American Hospital Association
- American Medical Association
- Association of American Medical Colleges
- Council of Medical Specialty Societies

Each member organization nominates four individuals to the ACGME's Board of Directors. In addition, the Board of Directors includes three public representatives, two resident representatives, and the chair of the Council of Review Committee Chairs. A representative for the federal government also serves on the Board in a non-voting capacity.

American Board of Medical Specialties (ABMS®)

Note: See page 126 for more information.

A nonprofit organization of 24 approved medical specialty boards. Its mission is to maintain and improve the quality of medical care by helping its member boards develop and use professional and educational standards for the evaluation and certification of physician specialists. The certification of physicians provides assurance to the public that a physician specialist certified by an ABMS member board has successfully completed an approved educational program and an evaluation process that assesses the knowledge, skills, and experience required to provide quality patient care in that specialty. Medical specialty board certification is an additional process to receiving a medical degree, completing residency training, and receiving a license to practice medicine.

Boards and certification

Note: See page 126 for more information.

Each medical specialty (as defined by the ABMS) has its own unique Board examination process. This process is voluntary and is intended to assure the public that a certified medical specialist has successfully completed an approved educational program and an evaluation including an examination process designed to assess the knowledge, experience, and skills requisite to the provision of high-quality patient care in that specialty.

General board certification is the first certification awarded by an ABMS member board to approved candidates who meet the requirements for certification in a specified field of medical practice.

Subspecialty board certification is conferred by one or more ABMS member boards in a component of a specialty or subspecialty. It is conferred only to certified medical specialists who have been certified by one or more member boards in an area of general certification.

Some ABMS member boards also issue *certificates of added qualifications* or *certificates of special qualifications.* (Source: ABMS)

Also see "Maintenance of Certification."

Clerkship

Note: See page 33 for more information.

Clinical education provided to medical students. Table 10 contains information on clerkship regulations of state medical boards.

Clinical Skills Assessment (CSA)

A 1-day exam, formerly administered by the ECFMG, that required examinees to demonstrate both clinical proficiency and spoken English language proficiency. Step 2 Clinical Skills (Step 2 CS) of the USMLE is the exam currently administered that satisfies the clinical skills requirement for ECFMG Certification.

Also see "Step 2 CS," page 104.

Comprehensive Osteopathic Medical Licensing Examination (COMLEX)

Note: See page 101 for more information.

A three-level examination initiated in 1995 by the National Board of Osteopathic Medical Examiners to replace the former three-part NBOME examination series and to better assist the state licensing boards in measuring the knowledge required by today's physicians.

The COMLEX program is designed to assess the osteopathic medical knowledge considered essential for osteopathic generalist physicians to practice medicine without supervision. COMLEX is constructed in the context of medical problem solving, which involves clinical presentations and physician tasks.

ECFMG number

Note: See page 104 for more information.

The number assigned by the Educational Commission for Foreign Medical Graduates (ECFMG) to each international medical graduate (IMG) who applies for certification from ECFMG. Almost all graduates of foreign medical schools must have an ECFMG Certificate to participate in graduate medical education in the United States.

Educational Commission for Foreign Medical Graduates (ECFMG)

Note: See page 104 for more information.

A nonprofit organization that assesses the readiness of graduates of foreign medical schools to enter residency programs in the United States accredited by the Accreditation Council for Graduate Medical Education (ACGME).

ECFMG certification provides assurance to directors of ACGME-accredited residency programs, and to the people of the United States, that graduates of foreign medical schools have met minimum standards of eligibility required to enter such programs. This certification does not guarantee that such graduates will be accepted into these programs in the United States, since the number of applicants frequently exceeds the number of positions available.

ECFMG certification is also a prerequisite required by most states for licensure to practice medicine in the United States and is one of the eligibility requirements to take Step 3 of the United States Medical Licensing Examination (USMLE).

Endorsement, licensure

Note: See page 11 for more information.

A process through which a state issues an unrestricted license to practice medicine to an individual who holds a valid and unrestricted license in another jurisdiction. Licensure endorsement is generally based on documentation of successfully completing approved examinations, authentication of required core documents, and completion of any additional requirements assessing the applicant's fitness to practice medicine in the new jurisdiction. Previously referred to as "reciprocity."

Fellow

A. A physician in an ACGME-accredited program that is beyond the requirements for eligibility for first board certification in the discipline. Such physicians may also be termed "resident" as well. Other uses of the term "fellow" require modifiers for precision and clarity, e.g., "research fellow."
   Also see "Resident or resident physician."

B. A physician who has demonstrated outstanding achievements in medicine, usually within a given medical specialty society. Typical criteria for fellowship in a specialty society include years of membership, years as a practitioner in the specialty, and professional recognition by peers.

Federation Licensing Examination (FLEX)

Note: See page 11 for more information.

Originally introduced in 1968 and subsequently enhanced and modified in 1985, this examination was administered for the last time in December 1993. In 1994, the United States Medical Licensing Examination (USMLE) was fully implemented. Some candidates for licensure may have a combination of scores from FLEX and USMLE. *Also see "United States Medical Licensing Examination."*

Federation of State Medical Boards (FSMB)

Note: See page 96 for more information.

A nonprofit organization whose membership comprises the allopathic, osteopathic, and composite medical licensing boards of all the states, the District of Columbia, Guam, Puerto Rico, and the Virgin Islands. Its primary responsibility is to protect the public through the regulation of physicians and other health care providers. It serves as a liaison, advocate, and information source to the public, health care organizations, and state, national, and international authorities. The FSMB promotes high standards for physician licensure and practice and assists and supports state medical boards collectively and individually in the regulation of medical practice and in their role of public protection.

Fifth Pathway

Note: See page 28 for more information.

One of several ways that individuals who obtain their undergraduate medical education abroad can enter GME in the United States. The Fifth Pathway is a period of supervised clinical training for students who obtained their premedical education in the United States, received undergraduate medical education abroad, and passed Step 1 of the United States Medical Licensing Examination. After these students successfully complete a year of clinical training sponsored by a US medical school accredited by the Liaison Committee on Medical Education (LCME) and pass USMLE Step 2, they receive a Fifth Pathway certificate and become eligible for an ACGME-accredited residency as an international medical graduate. *Note:* The Fifth Pathway was being discontinued as of June 30, 2009.

FLEX Weighted Average (FWA)

Note: See page 11 for more information.

All states currently require a minimum passing score of 75 on each component of the post-1985 two-part FLEX; the resulting number composes the Federation Licensing Examination (FLEX) Weighted Average.

Initial license

Note: See page 84 for more information.

The first ever full and unrestricted license a physician receives in his/her medical career. Some medical boards interpret "initial license" as a physician's first license in their particular states (although the physician could already have been licensed in other states). This publication does not use the term in this sense.

Intern

No longer used by the AMA or ACGME. Historically, "intern" was used to designate individuals in the first post-MD year of hospital training; less commonly, it designated individuals in the first year of any residency program. Since 1975, the AMA's *Graduate Medical Education Directory* and the ACGME have used "resident," "resident physician," or "fellow" to designate all individuals in ACGME-accredited programs. *Also see "Resident or resident physician" and "Fellow."*

International medical graduate (IMG)

A graduate from a medical school outside of the United States and Canada. Formerly referred to as "foreign medical graduate" (FMG).

Liaison Committee on Medical Education (LCME)

The body that accredits educational programs in the United States and Canada leading to the MD degree. The American Osteopathic Association (AOA) accredits educational programs leading to the doctor of osteopathy (DO) degree.

Licensure

The process by which a state or jurisdiction of the United States admits physicians to the practice of medicine. Licensure ensures that practicing physicians have appropriate education and training and that they abide by recognized standards of professional conduct while serving their patients. Candidates for first licensure must complete a rigorous examination designed to assess a physician's ability to apply knowledge, concepts, and principles that are important in health and disease and that constitute the basis of safe and effective patient care. All applicants must submit proof of medical education and training and provide details about their work history. Finally, applicants may have to reveal information regarding past medical history (including the use of habit-forming drugs and emotional or mental illness), arrests, and convictions. *Also see "Limited license" and "Reregistration."*

Limited license

Note: See page 57 for more information.

Issued by state medical boards to resident physicians in graduate medical education (GME) programs within their jurisdictions. Physicians do not receive a full and unrestricted license until completion of GME and fulfillment of other licensure requirements in a given jurisdiction.

Maintenance of Certification

Note: See page 126 for more information.

To better evaluate the competence of physician specialists throughout their careers, ABMS Member Boards are moving from "recertification" to a more comprehensive plan called "maintenance of certification." Where recertification programs evaluate physicians every 7 to 10 years, primarily by a written examination, Maintenance of Certification© is an in-depth program that will be continuous and relevant to practice. A key component of this program is the evaluation of physician practice performance, including six core competencies (patient care, medical knowledge, interpersonal and communication skills, professionalism, practice-based learning and improvement, and systems-based practice).

Medical Practice Act

A statute of a US state or jurisdiction that outlines the practice of medicine and the responsibility of the medical board to regulate that practice. The primary responsibility and obligation of a state medical board is to protect the public through proper licensing and regulation of physicians and, in some jurisdictions, other health care professionals. *Also see "Unprofessional conduct."*

National Board of Medical Examiners (NBME)

Note: See page 99 for more information.

A nonprofit, independent organization that prepares and administers medical qualifying examinations, either independently or jointly with other organizations. Legal agencies governing the practice of medicine within each US state or jurisdiction may grant a license without further examination for those physicians who have successfully completed such examinations and met other requirements.

Currently, the NBME administers USMLE Steps 1 and 2 to students and graduates of US and Canadian medical and osteopathic schools accredited by the Liaison Committee on Medical Education or the American Osteopathic Association.

National Board of Osteopathic Medical Examiners (NBOME)

Note: See page 101 for more information.

A not-for-profit corporation serving the public and state licensing agencies by administering examinations testing the medical knowledge of those who seek to practice as osteopathic physicians.

The NBOME examinations have been the primary pathway by which osteopathic physicians have applied for licensure to practice osteopathic medicine. A passing score on these examinations verifies a student's adequacy of medical knowledge for practicing osteopathic medicine.

Reregistration

Note: See page 53 for more information.

After physicians are licensed in a state or jurisdiction, they must reregister periodically to continue their active status. During this reregistration process, physicians are required to demonstrate that they have maintained acceptable standards of ethics and medical practice and have not engaged in improper conduct. In many states, physicians must also show that they have completed a set number of hours of continuing medical education.

Resident or resident physician

Any individual at any level in an ACGME-accredited GME program, including subspecialty programs. Local usage might refer to these individuals as interns, house officers, house staff, trainees, fellows, or other comparable terminology. Beginning in 2000, the ACGME has used the term "fellow" to denote physicians in subspecialty programs (vs residents in specialty programs) or in GME programs that are beyond the requirements for eligibility for first board certification in the discipline.

Also see "Fellow."

Special Purpose Examination (SPEX)

Note: See page 98 for more information.

This 1-day, computer-administered examination, with approximately 420 multiple-choice questions, assesses primary care medical knowledge and skills. It does not include questions specific to a particular specialty or subspecialty. The SPEX is used to assess physicians who have held a valid, unrestricted license in a US or Canadian jurisdiction who are:

- Required by the state medical board to demonstrate current medical knowledge
- Seeking endorsement licensure some years beyond initial examination
- Seeking license reinstatement after a period of professional inactivity

Physicians holding a valid, unrestricted license may also apply for SPEX, independent of any request or approval from a medical licensing board.

Specialty

A medical specialty is a defined area of medical practice that connotes special knowledge and ability resulting from specialized effort and training in the special field. (Source: ABMS)

Also see "Subspecialty."

Step 2 CS

The Clinical Skills component of USMLE Step 2, in tandem with the Clinical Knowledge component (Step 2 CK), became a part of Step 2 in June 2004. Step 2 assesses whether medical school students and graduates can understand and apply the knowledge, skills, and understanding of clinical science considered essential for the provision of patient care under supervision and includes emphasis on health promotion and disease prevention. The inclusion of Step 2 in the USMLE sequence is intended to ensure that due attention is devoted to principles of clinical sciences and basic patient-centered skills that provide the foundation for safe and competent medical practice.

Subspecialty

A medical subspecialty is an identifiable component of a specialty to which a practicing physician may devote a significant proportion of time. Practice in the subspecialty follows special educational experience in addition to that required for general certification. (*Note:* Two different specialty fields may include two or more similar subspecialty areas, e.g., sports medicine as a subspecialty of emergency medicine and family practice. In these cases the identified subspecialty area might use the same title and equivalent educational standards.) (Source: ABMS)

Also see "Specialty."

Telemedicine

Note: See page 77 for more information.

Telemedicine is the delivery of health care services via electronic means from a health care provider in one location to a patient in another. Applications that fall under this definition include the transfer of medical images, such as pathology slides or radiographs, interactive video consultations between patient and provider or between primary care and specialty care physicians, and mental health consultations.

Unprofessional conduct

Although laws vary from one jurisdiction to the next, the Medical Practice Acts in force in most US jurisdictions would define unprofessional conduct as including:

- Physical abuse of a patient
- Inadequate recordkeeping
- Not recognizing or acting on common symptoms
- Prescribing drugs in excessive amounts or without legitimate reason
- Impaired ability to practice due to addiction or physical or mental illness
- Failing to meet continuing medical education requirements
- Performing duties beyond the scope of a license
- Dishonesty
- Conviction of a felony
- Delegating the practice of medicine to an unlicensed individual

Unprofessional conduct would not include minor disagreements or poor customer service.

United States Medical Licensing Examination (USMLE)

Note: See page 90 for more information.

This three-step examination for US medical licensure provides a common evaluation system for applicants. The USMLE program is governed by a composite committee of representatives from the Federation of State Medical Boards (FSMB), the National Board of Medical Examiners (NBME), the Educational Commission for Foreign Medical Graduates (ECFMG), and the public.

Results of the USMLE are reported to state medical boards for use in granting the initial license to practice medicine. Each medical licensing authority requires, as part of its licensing processes, successful completion of an examination or other certification demonstrating qualification for licensure.

The USMLE replaced FLEX and the certifying examination of the NBME, as well as the Foreign Medical Graduate Examination in the Medical Sciences (FMGEMS), which was formerly used by the ECFMG for certification purposes. Steps 1 and 2 of the USMLE are used as the examination for ECFMG certification. These two steps are also used for promotion and graduation in some US medical schools.

Appendix E

AMA Policy on Medical Licensure

The AMA has a number of policy statements concerning medical licensure. Following is representative AMA policy in this regard, as found in the AMA's Policy Finder, using a search for the term "licensure" (returning 103 results total) in June 2009.

The H prefix indicates that the policy was developed by the AMA House of Delegates; the D prefix indicates that the policy is a directive from the AMA House for the Association to take a specific action.

The number assigned to a policy indicates the topic addressed by the policy. For example, House policies coded between H-255.001 and H-255.999 all relate to the topic of "International Medical Graduates."

Contents

D-255.000 International Medical Graduates

D-275.000 Licensure and Discipline

D-480.000 Technology

Guidance for Physicians on Internet Prescribing H-120.949

Our AMA provides the following guidance for physicians on the appropriate use of the Internet in prescribing medications:

(a) Criteria for an acceptable patient (clinical) encounter and follow-up:
Physicians who prescribe medications via the Internet shall establish, or have established, a valid patient-physician relationship, including, but not limited to, the following components. The physician shall: (i) obtain a reliable medical history and perform a physical examination of the patient, adequate to establish the diagnosis for which the drug is being prescribed and to identify underlying conditions and/or contraindications to the treatment recommended/provided; (ii) have sufficient dialogue with the patient regarding treatment options and the risks and benefits of treatment(s); (iii) as appropriate, follow up with the patient to assess the therapeutic outcome; (iv) maintain a contemporaneous medical record that is readily available to the patient and, subject to the patient's consent, to his or her other health care professionals; and (v) include the electronic prescription information as part of the patient medical record. Exceptions to the above criteria exist in the following specific instances: treatment provided in consultation with another physician who has an ongoing professional relationship with the patient, and who has agreed to supervise the patient's treatment, including use of any prescribed medications; and on-call or cross-coverage situations.

(b) Licensure
Physicians who prescribe medications via the Internet across state lines, without physically being located in the state(s) where the patient (clinical) encounter(s) occurs, must possess appropriate licensure in all jurisdictions where patients reside. An exception to this requirement is when the clinical encounter with the patient, as described in recommendation 1(a) above, occurs in the state where the physician is licensed and his or her practice is located, and the state where the patient resides allows electronic prescriptions from out-of-state prescribers.

(c) Security of patient information
Physicians who prescribe via the Internet should transmit prescriptions over a secure network (i.e., provisions for password protection, encrypted electronic prescriptions, or other reliable authentication techniques [e.g., AMA Internet ID]) in order to protect patient privacy.

(d) Disclosure of identifying information on web sites
Physicians who practice medicine via the Internet, including prescribing, should clearly disclose physician-identifying information on the web site, including (but not necessarily limited to) name, practice location (address and contact information), and all states in which licensure is held. Posting of actual physicians' license numbers (e.g., the DEA number) is unnecessary.

(e) Liability exposure
Physicians should be aware that they may increase their liability exposure by prescribing medications to individuals solely through online interactions (e.g., online questionnaire or online consultation).

(BOT Rep. 7, A-03; Reaffirmed: BOT Rep. 3, I-04; Reaffirmed: Sub. Res. 522, A-05)

Supply and Distribution of Health Professionals H-200.987

1. Licensure, certification and accreditation should not be used for the purpose of regulating the supply of health professionals.

2. Health professions' curricula should emphasize the needs of underserved populations, including the poor, minorities, the chronically ill and disabled, and the geographically isolated. Decisions regarding the financing of health professions education should be based in part on the data and analyses of the national consortium on the supply and distribution of health professionals.

(BOT Rep. NN, A-87; Reaffirmed: Sunset Report, I-97; Reaffirmation A-01; Modified: CME Rep. 2, I-03)

Equality in Licensure and Reciprocity
H-255.982

Our AMA

1. Reaffirms its policy that it is inappropriate to discriminate against any physician because of national origin or geographical location of medical education

2. Continues to recognize the right and responsibility of states and territories to determine the qualifications of individuals applying for licensure to practice medicine within their respective jurisdiction

3. Supports the development and distribution of model legislation to encourage states to amend their Medical Practice Acts to provide that graduates of foreign medical schools shall meet the same requirements for licensure by endorsement as graduates of accredited US and Canadian schools.

(Res. 69, A-89; Rescinded: Sunset Report, A-00; Restored: CME Rep. 3, A-02; Reaffirmed: CME Rep. 7, A-04; Reaffirmed in lieu of Res. 320, A-04)

Graduates of Non-United States Medical Schools
H-255.983

The AMA continues to support the policy that all physicians and medical students should be evaluated for purposes of entry into graduate medical education programs, licensure, and hospital medical staff privileges on the basis of their individual qualifications, skills, and character.

(Sub. Res. 45, A-88; Reaffirmed by Res. 311, A-96; Reaffirmed: CMS Rep. 10, A-03; Reaffirmed: CME Rep. 1, I-03; Reaffirmed: CME Rep. 7, A-04; Reaffirmed: Sub. Res. 314, A-04)

Report of the Ad Hoc Committee on Foreign Medical Graduates
H-255.988

1. The AMA reaffirms its support of current US visa and immigration requirements applicable to foreign national physicians who are graduates of medical schools other than those in the United States and Canada.

2. The AMA continues to support current regulations governing the issuance of exchange visitor visas to foreign national IMGs, including the requirements for successful completion of the USMLE.

3. The AMA reaffirms its policy that the US and Canada medical schools be accredited by a nongovernmental accrediting body.

4. The AMA continues to support cooperation in the collection and analysis of information on medical schools in nations other than the US and Canada.

5. The AMA supports continued cooperation with the ECFMG and other appropriate organizations to disseminate information to prospective and current students in foreign medical schools.

6. The AMA continues to support working with the ECFMG and other appropriate organizations in developing effective methods to evaluate the clinical skills of IMGs.

7. The AMA strongly supports the policy that the core clinical curriculum of a foreign medical school should be provided by that school and that US hospitals should not provide substitute core clinical experience for students attending a foreign medical school.

8. The AMA continues to support working with the Accreditation Council for Graduate Medical Education (ACGME) and the Federation of State Medical Boards (FSMB) to assure that institutions offering accredited residencies, residency program directors, and US licensing authorities do not deviate from established standards when evaluating graduates of foreign medical schools.

9. The AMA, in cooperation with the ACGME and the FSMB, supports only those modifications in established graduate medical education or licensing standards designed to enhance the quality of medical education and patient care.

10. The AMA continues to support the activities of the ECFMG related to verification of education credentials and testing of IMGs.

11. Special consideration should be given to the limited number of IMGs who are refugees from foreign governments that refuse to provide pertinent information usually required to establish eligibility for residency training or licensure.

12. The AMA reaffirms its existing policy supporting the use of accreditation standards to enhance the quality of patient care and medical education. Also the AMA opposes the use of such standards for purposes of regulating physician manpower.

13. AMA representatives to the ACGME, residency review committees and to the ECFMG should support AMA policy opposing discrimination. In particular, these

AMA representatives should emphasize that AMA policy does not prohibit the appointment of qualified graduates of foreign medical schools to residency training programs.

14. The AMA strongly reaffirms existing policy urging the US licensing authorities to focus on the individual academic and personal achievements when evaluating IMGs for the purposes of licensure. More effective methods for evaluating the quality of the undergraduate medical education of IMGs should be pursued and, when available, the results should be a part of the determination of eligibility for licensure.

15. The AMA reaffirms its support for the requirement that all medical school graduates complete at least one year of graduate medical education in an accredited US program in order to qualify for full and unrestricted licensure.

16. The AMA supports continued monitoring of the effectiveness of the Fifth Pathway program, including to the degree possible any measurable impact of the program on enrollments in Caribbean and Central American medical schools.

17. The AMA reaffirms and supports publicizing existing policy concerning the granting of staff and clinical privileges in hospitals and other health facilities.

18. The AMA reaffirms its support of the participation of all physicians, including graduates of foreign as well as US and Canadian medical schools, in organized medicine.

19. The AMA encourages the constituent medical societies to support qualified IMGs for nominations to AMA committees and councils.

20. The AMA supports studying the feasibility of conducting peer-to-peer membership recruitment efforts aimed at IMGs who are not AMA members.

21. The AMA is committed to using its existing publications to highlight policies and activities of interest to IMGs, stressing the common concerns of all physicians.

22. The AMA supports demonstrating its interests in issues related to IMGs by publicizing its many relevant resources to all physicians, especially to nonmember IMGs.

23. The AMA supports expansion of its efforts to prepare and disseminate information about requirements for admission to accredited residency programs, the availability of positions, and the problems of becoming licensed and entering full and unrestricted medical practice in the US that face IMGs. This information should be addressed to college students, high school and college advisors, and students in foreign medical schools.

24. The AMA continues to recognize the common aims and goals of all physicians, particularly those practicing in the US, and supports making every effort to include all physicians who are permanent residents of the US in the mainstream of American medicine.

25. The AMA is committed to identifying and publicizing resources within the AMA that will respond to inquiries from IMGs.

26. The AMA is committed to providing leadership to promote the international exchange of medical knowledge as well as cultural understanding between the US and other nations.

27. The AMA urges institutions that sponsor exchange visitor programs in medical education, clinical medicine and public health to tailor programs for the individual visiting scholar that will meet the needs of the scholar, the institution, and the nation to which he will return.

28. The AMA is committed to informing foreign national IMGs that the availability of training and practice opportunities in the US is limited by the availability of fiscal and human resources to maintain the quality of medical education and patient care in the US.

(BOT Rep. Z, A-86; Reaffirmed: Res. 312, I-93; Modified: CME Rep. 2, A-03)

Discrimination Against Physicians H-255.992

Our AMA:

1. Believes that the quality of a physician's medical education is an appropriate consideration in the recruitment and licensure of physicians and discrimination against physicians on the basis of the country in which they completed their medical education is inappropriate

2. Affirms that the residency application process should be free of discrimination, including discrimination arising from the electronic submission of applications.

(Sub. Res. 44, A-85; Reaffirmed: CLRPD Rep. 2, I-95; Appended: Sub. Res. 305 and Reaffirmation A-00)

Physician Exemption from Medical School Standards and Performance Evaluation Requirements H-255.994

1. The AMA recommends to medical licensing boards that those physicians who are foreign medical graduates currently duly licensed by any licensing jurisdiction in the US should not be denied endorsement of their licenses, or denied admission to reexamination when this is required by law, solely because they are unable to provide documentation of graduation from a school meeting "equivalent standards and performance evaluation requirements" to those of programs accredited by the Liaison Committee on Medical Education.

2. The AMA encourages licensing boards, in reviewing applications for licensure endorsement, to take into account a physician's ethical standards and his or her having practiced medicine of an acceptable quality.

(Sub. Res. 108, A-83; Reaffirmed: CLRPD Rep. 1, I-93; Reaffirmed: CME Rep. 2, A-05)

International Medical Graduates H-255.995

The AMA believes that reduced requirements for licensure should not be applied under any circumstances to graduates of foreign medical schools.

(Res. 23, A-82; Reaffirmed: CLRPD Rep. A, I-92; Modified: CME Rep. 5, A-04)

Arbitrary Exclusion of International Medical Schools Which Impacts Physician Licensure H-275.928

Our AMA opposes the practice by state medical boards of creating arbitrary and non criterion-based lists of approved or unapproved international medical schools.

(Res. 310, A-05)

Additions to United States Medical Licensure Examination and Comprehensive Osteopathic Medical Licensure Examination H-275.929

Our AMA opposes additions to the United States Medical Licensing Examination and Comprehensive Osteopathic Medical Licensure Examination that lack predictive validity for future performance as a physician.

(Res. 308, A-04)

Internal Medicine Board Certification Report—Interim Report H-275.932

Our AMA opposes the use of recertification or Maintenance of Certification (MOC) as a condition of employment, licensure or reimbursement.

(CME Rep. 7, A-02)

Alternatives to the Federation of State Medical Boards' Recommendations on Licensure H-275.934

Our AMA adopts the following principles:

1. Ideally, all medical students should successfully complete Steps 1 and 2 of the United States Medical Licensing Examination (USMLE) or Parts 1 and 2 of the Comprehensive Osteopathic Medical Licensing Examination (COMLEX) prior to entry into residency training. At a minimum, individuals entering residency training must have successfully completed Step 1 of the USMLE or Part 1 of COMLEX. There should be provision made for students who have not completed Step 2 of the USMLE or Part 2 of the COMLEX to do so during the first year of residency training.

2. All applicants for full and unrestricted licensure, whether graduates of US medical schools or international medical graduates, must have completed one year of accredited graduate medical education (GME) in the US, have passed all licensing examinations (USMLE or COMLEX), and must be certified by their residency program director as ready to advance to the next year of GME and to obtain a full and unrestricted license to practice medicine. The candidate for licensure should have had education that provided exposure to general medical content.

3. There should be a training permit/educational license for all resident physicians who do not yet have a full and unrestricted license to practice medicine. To be eligible for an initial training permit/educational license, the resident must have completed Step 1 of the USMLE or Part 1 of COMLEX.

4. Residency program directors shall report only those actions to state medical licensing boards that are reported for all licensed physicians.

5. Residency program directors should receive training to ensure that they understand the process for taking disciplinary action against resident physicians, and are aware of procedures for dismissal of residents and for due process. This requirement for residency program directors should be enforced through Accreditation Council for Graduate Medical Education accreditation requirements.

6. There should be no reporting of actions against medical students to state medical licensing boards.

7. Medical schools are responsible for identifying and remediating and/or disciplining medical student unprofessional behavior, problems with substance abuse, and other behavioral problems. as well as gaps in student knowledge and skills.

8. The Dean's Letter of Evaluation should be strengthened and standardized, to serve as a better source of information to residency programs about applicants.

(CME Rep. 8, A-99; Reaffirmed: CME Rep. 4, I-01)

Licensure of IMGs
H-275.935

Our AMA asks the Federation of State Medical Boards to ask all the state licensing boards to adopt a uniform standard governing the allowed number of administrations of the licensure examinations.

(Res. 314, A-99)

Mechanisms to Measure Physician Competency
H-275.936

Our AMA (1) reviews and proposes improvements for assuring continued physician competence, including but not limited to performance indicators, board certification and recertification, professional experience, continuing medical education, and teaching experience; and (2) opposes the development and/or use of "Medical Competency Examination" and establishment of oversight boards for current state medical boards as proposed in the fall 1998 Report on Professional Licensure of the Pew Health Professions Commission, as an additional measure of physician competency.

(Res. 320, I-98; Amended: Res. 817, A-99; Reaffirmed: CME Rep. 7, A-02; Reaffirmed: CME Rep. 7, A-07)

USMLE Part III and Licensure
H-275.938

Our AMA will lobby the Federation of State Medical Boards to discourage states from linking mandatory application for licensure with application to take the USMLE Part III.

(Res. 325, A-98)

Out-of-State Residents in Training and State Licensing Board Requirements for Temporary Licenses
H-275.941

The AMA will work with the Federation of State Medical Boards (FSMB) to facilitate a timely process so that residents in a training program can meet the licensure requirements to avail themselves of opportunities for educational experiences in states other than that of their primary program location.

(Sub. Res. 301, A-97; Reaffirmed: CME Rep. 2, A-07)

Self-Incriminating Questions on Applications for Licensure and Specialty Boards
H-275.945

The AMA will:

1. Encourage the Federation of State Medical Boards and its constituent members to develop uniform definitions and nomenclature for use in licensing and disciplinary proceedings to better facilitate the sharing of information

2. Seek clarification of the application of the Americans with Disabilities Act to the actions of medical licensing and medical specialty boards

3. Until the applicability and scope of the Americans with Disabilities Act are clarified, will encourage the American Board of Medical Specialties and the Federation of State Medical Boards and their constituent members to advise physicians of the rationale behind inquiries on mental illness, substance abuse or physical disabilities in materials used in the licensure, reregistration, and certification processes when such questions are asked.

(BOT Rep. 1, I-933; CME Rep. 10 - I-94; Reaffirmed: CME Rep. 2, A-04)

Board Certification
H-275.950

Our AMA

1. Reaffirms its opposition to the use of board certification as a requirement for licensure or reimbursement

2. Seeks an amendment to the new Medicaid rules that would delete the use of board certification as a requirement for reimbursement and would address the exclusion of internal medicine, emergency medicine, and other specialties.

(Res. 143, A-92; ; Reaffirmed by Res. 108, A-98; Reaffirmation A-00)

Mandatory Acceptance of Patient's Group Plan
H-275.951

It is the policy of the AMA that the sole purpose of medical licensure is to assure the competence of physicians to practice medicine.

(Sub. Res. 111, I-91; Modified: Sunset Report, I-01)

Physician Licensure Legislation
H-275.955

Our AMA (1) reaffirms its policies opposing discrimination against physicians on the basis of being a graduate of a foreign medical school and supports state and territory responsibility for admitting physicians to practice; and (2) reaffirms earlier policy urging licensing jurisdictions to adopt laws and rules facilitating the movement of physicians between states, to move toward uniformity in requirements for the endorsement of licenses to practice medicine, and to base endorsement of medical licenses on an assessment of competence rather than on passing a written examination of cognitive knowledge.

(CME Rep. B, A-90; Reaffirmation A-00)

Demonstration of Clinical Competence
H-275.956

It is the policy of the AMA to

1. Support continued efforts to develop and validate methods for assessment of clinical skills

2. Continue its participation in the development and testing of methods for clinical skills assessment

3. Recognize that clinical skills assessment is best performed using a rigorous and consistent examination administered by medical schools and should not be used for licensure of graduates of Liaison Committee on Medical Education (LCME)- and American Osteopathic Association (AOA)-accredited medical schools or of Educational Commission for Foreign Medical Graduates (ECFMG)-certified physicians.

(CME Rep. E, A-90; Reaffirmed: CME Rep. 5, A-99; Modified: Sub. Res. 821, I-02; Modified: CME Rep. 1, I-03)

Postgraduate Training Requirements for Obtaining Permanent Medical Licensure
H-275.960

Our AMA continues to oppose lengthy residency training requirements for licensure.

(CME Rep. A, I-89; Reaffirmed: Sunset Report, A-00)

Proposed Single Examination for Licensure
H-275.962

Our AMA:

1. Endorses the concept of a single examination for medical licensure

2. Urges the NBME and the FSMB to place responsibility for developing Steps I and II of the new single examination for licensure with the faculty of US medical schools working through the NBME

3. Continues its vigorous support of the LCME and its accreditation of medical schools and supports monitoring the impact of a single examination on the effectiveness of the LCME

4. Urges the NBME and the FSMB to establish a high standard for passing the examination

5. Strongly recommends and supports actively pursuing efforts to assure that the standard for passing be criterion-based; that is, that passing the examination indicate a degree of knowledge acceptable for practicing medicine

6. Urges that appointing graduates of LCME-accredited medical schools to accredited residency training not be dependent on their passing Steps I and II or the single examination for licensure.

(CME Rep. B, I-89; Reaffirmed: Sunset Report, A-00)

Mandatory Medicare Assignment or Determination of Fee Levels
H-275.963

Our AMA supports federal legislation that would prohibit states from enacting legislation to require that acceptance of Medicare assignment or the Medicare allowance of reimbursement be a condition of medical licensure, or used in determinations of unprofessional conduct, or made effectively mandatory in any other fashion.

(Sub Res. 75, A-89; Reaffirmed: Sunset Report, A-00)

Licensure by Endorsement
H-275.967

The AMA opposes national legislation which would mandate licensing reciprocity by all state licensing authorities.

(Res. 42, A-88; Reaffirmed: Sunset Report, I-98)

Licensure Confidentiality
H-275.970

The AMA

1. Encourages specialty boards, hospitals, and other organizations involved in credentialing, as well as state licensing boards, to take all necessary steps to assure the confidentiality of information contained on application forms for credentials

2. Encourages boards to include in application forms only requests for information that can reasonably be related to medical practice

3. Encourages state licensing boards to exclude from license application forms information that refers to psychoanalysis, counseling, or psychotherapy required or undertaken as part of medical training

4. Encourages state medical societies and specialty societies to join with the AMA in efforts to change statutes and regulations to provide needed confidentiality for information collected by licensing boards

5. Encourages state licensing boards to require that, if an applicant has had psychiatric treatment, the physician who has provided the treatment submit to the board an official statement that the applicant's current state of health does not interfere with his or her ability to practice medicine.

(CME Rep. B, A-88; Reaffirmed: BOT Rep. 1, I-933; CME Rep. 10 - I-94; Reaffirmed: CME Rep. 2, A-04)

State Control of Qualifications for Medical Licensure
H-275.973

1. The AMA firmly opposes the imposition of federally mandated restrictions on the ability of individual states to determine the qualifications of physician candidates for licensure by endorsement.

2. The AMA actively opposes the enactment of any legislation introduced in Congress that promotes these objectives.

(Res. 84, I-87; Reaffirmed: Sunset Report, I-97; Reaffirmed: CME Rep. 2, A-07)

Qualifications of Health Professionals
H-275.975

(1) Private certifying organizations should be encouraged to continue certification programs for all health professionals and to communicate to the public the qualifications and standards they require for certification. Decisions concerning recertification should be made by the certifying organizations. (2) Working with state licensing and certifying boards, health care professions should use the results of quality assurance activities to ensure that substandard practitioner behavior is dealt with in a professional and timely manner. Licensure and disciplinary boards, in cooperation with their respective professional and occupational associations, should be encouraged to work to identify "deficient" health care professionals.

(BOT Rep. NN, A-87; Reaffirmed: Sunset Report, I-97; Reaffirmed: CME Rep. 2, A-07)

Boundaries of Practice for Health Professionals
H-275.976

(1) The health professional who coordinates an individual's health care has an ethical responsibility to ensure that the services required by an individual patient are provided by a professional whose basic competence and current performance are suited to render those services safely and effectively. In addition, patients also have a responsibility for maintaining coordination and continuity of their own health care. (2) As a supplement to strengthen state licensure of health professionals, standard-setting and self-regulatory competency assurance programs should be conducted by health professions associations, certifying and accrediting agencies, and health care facilities.

(BOT Rep. NN, A-87; Reaffirmed: Sunset Report, I-97

Medical Licensure
H-275.978

The AMA:

1. Urges directors of accredited residency training programs to certify the clinical competence of graduates of foreign medical schools after completion of the first year of residency training; however, program directors must not provide certification until they are satisfied that the resident is clinically competent

2. Encourages licensing boards to require a certificate of competence for full and unrestricted licensure

3. Urges licensing boards to review the details of application for initial licensure to assure that procedures are not unnecessarily cumbersome and that inappropriate information is not required. Accurate identification of documents and applicants is critical. It is recommended that boards continue to work cooperatively with the Federation of State Medical Boards to these ends

4. Will continue to provide information to licensing boards and other health organizations in an effort to prevent the use of fraudulent credentials for entry to medical practice

5. Urges those licensing boards that have not done so to develop regulations permitting the issuance of special purpose licenses. It is recommended that these regulations permit special purpose licensure with the minimum of educational requirements consistent with protecting the health, safety and welfare of the public

6. Urges licensing boards, specialty boards, hospitals and their medical staffs, and other organizations that evaluate physician competence to inquire only into conditions which impair a physician's current ability to practice medicine (BOT Rep. I-93-13; CME Rep. 10 - I-94)

7. Urges licensing boards to maintain strict confidentiality of reported information

8. Urges that the evaluation of information collected by licensing boards be undertaken only by persons experienced in medical licensure and competent to make judgments about physician competence. It is recommended that decisions concerning medical competence and discipline be made with the participation of physician members of the board

9. Recommends that if confidential information is improperly released by a licensing board about a physician, the board take appropriate and immediate steps to correct any adverse consequences to the physician

10. Urges all physicians to participate in continuing medical education as a professional obligation

11. Urges licensing boards not to require mandatory reporting of continuing medical education as part of the process of reregistering the license to practice medicine

12. Opposes the use of written cognitive examinations of medical knowledge at the time of reregistration except when there is reason to believe that a physician's knowledge of medicine is deficient

13. Supports working with the Federation of State Medical Boards to develop mechanisms to evaluate the competence of physicians who do not have hospital privileges and who are not subject to peer review

14. Believes that licensing laws should relate only to requirements for admission to the practice of medicine and to assuring the continuing competence of physicians, and opposes efforts to achieve a variety of socioeconomic objectives through medical licensure regulation

15. Urges licensing jurisdictions to pass laws and adopt regulations facilitating the movement of licensed physicians between licensing jurisdictions; licensing jurisdictions should limit physician movement only for reasons related to protecting the health, safety and welfare of the public

16. Encourages the Federation of State Medical Boards and the individual medical licensing boards to continue to pursue the development of uniformity in the acceptance of examination scores on the Federation Licensing Examination and in other requirements for endorsement of medical licenses

17. Urges licensing boards not to place time limits on the acceptability of National Board certification or on scores on the United State Medical Licensing Examination for endorsement of licenses

18. Urges licensing boards to base endorsement on an assessment of physician competence and not on passing a written examination of cognitive ability, except in those instances when information collected by a licensing board indicates need for such an examination

19. Urges licensing boards to accept an initial license provided by another board to a graduate of a US medical school as proof of completion of acceptable medical education

20. Urges that documentation of graduation from a foreign medical school be maintained by boards providing an initial license, and that the documentation be provided on request to other licensing boards for review in connection with an application for licensure by endorsement

21. Urges licensing boards to consider the completion of specialty training and evidence of competent and honorable practice of medicine in reviewing applications for licensure by endorsement.

(CME Rep. A, A-87; Modified: Sunset Report, I-97; Reaffirmation A-04)

Medicare Reporting of Adverse Incidents in Hospitals to State Agencies
H-275.979

The AMA opposes the sharing of information generated through the Medicare utilization process or other institutional review with state licensure bodies until hospital quality assurance committees have been notified and given a reasonable time to respond.

(Res. 118, I-86; Reaffirmed: Sunset Report, I-96; Reaffirmed: CME Rep. 2, A-06)

Legislative Action
H-275.984

The AMA

1. Vigorously opposes legislation which mandates that, as a condition of licensure, physicians who treat Medicare beneficiaries must agree to charge or collect from Medicare beneficiaries no more than the Medicare allowed amount

2. Strongly affirms the policy that medical licensure should be determined by educational qualifications, professional competence, ethics and other appropriate factors necessary to assure professional character and fitness to practice

3. Opposes any law that compels either acceptance of Medicare assignment or acceptance of the Medicare allowed amount as payment in full as a condition of state licensure.

(Sub. Res. 117, I-85; Modified by CLRPD Rep. 2, I-95; Reaffirmed: BOT Rep. 12, A-05)

Graduate Medical Education Requirement for Medical Licensure
H-275.985

The AMA reaffirms its policy that all applicants for full and unrestricted licensure should be required to provide evidence of satisfactory completion of at least one year of an accredited program of graduate medical education in the US.

(CME Rep. E, I-85; Reaffirmed by CLRPD Rep. 2, I-95; Reaffirmed: CME Rep. 2, A-05)

Physician Participation in Third Party Payer Programs
H-275.994

The AMA opposes state laws making a physician's licensure contingent upon his providing services to Medicaid beneficiaries or any other specific category of patients.

(CMS Rep. N, A-81; Reaffirmed: CLRPD Rep. F, I-91; Reaffirmed by Res. 108, A-98)

Physician Competence
H-275.996

Our AMA:

1. Urges the American Board of Medical Specialties and its constituent boards to reconsider their positions regarding recertification as a mandatory requirement rather than as a voluntarily sought and achieved validation of excellence

2. Urges the Federation of State Medical Boards and its constituent state boards to reconsider and reverse their position urging and accepting specialty board certification as evidence of continuing competence for the purpose of re-registration of licensure

3. Favors continued efforts to improve voluntary continuing medical education programs, to maintain the peer review process within the profession, and to develop better techniques for establishing the necessary patient care data base.

(CME Rep. J, A-80; Reaffirmed: CLRPD Rep. B, I-90; Reaffirmed: Sunset Report, I-00; Reaffirmed: CME Rep. 7, A-02; Reaffirmed: CME Rep. 7, A-07)

Licensure by Specialty
H-275.997

Experience with licensure by specialty is too limited to determine what the long-range effects will be in the provision of timely, safe and comprehensive medical care. However, the AMA does not consider licensure by specialty to be desirable even in unusual cases.

(CME Rep. F, A-80; Reaffirmed: CLRPD Rep. B, I-90; Reaffirmed: Sunset Report, I-00)

Recommendations for Future Directions for Medical Education
H-295.995

(Note: Portion relevant to medical licensure excerpted below.)

The AMA supports the following recommendations relating to the future directions for medical education:

27. The AMA recommends to state licensing authorities that they require individual applicants, to be eligible to be licensed to practice medicine, to possess the degree of Doctor of Medicine or its equivalent from a school or program that meets the standards of the LCME or accredited by the American Osteopathic Association, or to demonstrate as individuals, comparable academic and personal achievements. All applicants for full and unrestricted licensure should provide evidence of the satisfactory completion of at least one year of an accredited program of graduate medical education in the US. Satisfactory completion should be based upon an assessment of the applicant's knowledge, problem-solving ability, and clinical skills in the general field of medicine. The AMA recommends to legislatures and governmental regulatory authorities that they not impose requirements for licensure that are so specific that they restrict the responsibility of medical educators to determine the content of undergraduate and graduate medical education.

30. US citizens should have access to factual information on the requirements for licensure and for reciprocity in the various jurisdictions, prerequisites for entry into graduate medical education programs, and other factors that should be considered before deciding to undertake the study of medicine in schools not accredited by the LCME.

(CME Rep. B, A-82; Amended: CLRPD Rep. A, I-92; Res. 331, I-95; Reaffirmed by Res. 322, A-97; Reaffirmation I-03; Modified: CME Rep. 7, A-05; Modified: CME Rep. 2, I-05)

Content-Specific CME Mandated for Licensure
H-300.953

1. The AMA, state medical societies, specialty societies, and other medical organizations should reaffirm that the medical profession alone has the responsibility for setting standards and determining curricula in continuing medical education.

2. State medical societies should establish avenues of communication with groups concerned with medical issues, so that these groups know that they have a place to go for discussion of issues and responding to problems.

3. State medical societies should periodically invite the various medical groups from within the state to discuss issues and priorities.

4. State medical societies in states which already have a content-specific CME requirement should consider appropriate ways of rescinding or amending the mandate.

(CME Rep. 6, A-96; Reaffirmed: CME Rep. 2, A-06)

Uniform Standards for Continuing Medical Education
H-300.969

The AMA (1) will continue its efforts to develop uniform standards for continuing medical education; and (2) will solicit input from all state medical associations, medical licensure boards, and national specialty organizations concerning the development of the most appropriate uniform standards for continuing medical education.

(Res. 313, A-92; Reaffirmed: CME Rep. 2, A-03; Reaffirmed in lieu of Res. 901, I-05)

Post-Licensure Assessment as a Condition for Physician Participation in Medicare
H-330.950

The AMA opposes proposals for periodic post-licensure assessment as a condition for physician participation in the Medicare program or other health-related entitlement program.

(Res. 231, I-93; Reaffirmed: BOT Rep. 28, A-03)

Resident Physician Licenses
H-405.966

The AMA supports the option of limited educational licenses in all states for resident physicians to provide care within their residency programs; and supports reduced licensure fees for resident physicians for participation solely in graduate medical education training programs when full medical licensure is required by a state.

(Sub. Res. 312, A-96; Reaffirmed: CME Rep. 2, A-06)

The Promotion of Quality Telemedicine
H-480.969

1. It is the policy of the AMA that medical boards of states and territories should require a full and unrestricted license in that state for the practice of telemedicine, unless there are other appropriate state-based licensing methods, with no differentiation by specialty, for physicians who wish to practice telemedicine in that state or territory. This license category should adhere to the following principles:
   (a) application to situations where there is a telemedical transmission of individual patient data from the patient's state that results in either (i) provision of a written or otherwise documented medical opinion used for diagnosis or treatment or (ii) rendering of treatment to a patient within the board's state;
   (b) exemption from such a licensure requirement for traditional informal physician-to-physician consultations ("curbside consultations") that are provided without expectation of compensation;
   (c) exemption from such a licensure requirement for telemedicine practiced across state lines in the event of an emergent or urgent circumstance, the definition of which for the purposes of telemedicine should show substantial deference to the judgment of the attending and consulting physicians as well as to the views of the patient; and
   (d) application requirements that are non-burdensome, issued in an expeditious manner, have fees no higher than necessary to cover the reasonable costs of administering this process, and that utilize principles of reciprocity with the licensure requirements of the state in which the physician in question practices.

2. The AMA urges the FSMB and individual states to recognize that a physician practicing certain forms of telemedicine (e.g., teleradiology) must sometimes perform necessary functions in the licensing state (e.g., interaction with patients, technologists, and

other physicians) and that the interstate telemedicine approach adopted must accommodate these essential quality-related functions.

3. The AMA urges national medical specialty societies to develop and implement practice parameters for telemedicine in conformance with Policy 410.973 (which identifies practice parameters as "educational tools"); Policy 410.987 (which identifies practice parameters as "strategies for patient management that are designed to assist physicians in clinical decision making," and states that a practice parameter developed by a particular specialty or specialties should not preclude the performance of the procedures or treatments addressed in that practice parameter by physicians who are not formally credentialed in that specialty or specialties); and Policy 410.996 (which states that physician groups representing all appropriate specialties and practice settings should be involved in developing practice parameters, particularly those which cross lines of disciplines or specialties).

(CME/CMS Rep., A-96; Amended: CME Rep. 7, A-99)

Evolving Impact of Telemedicine
H-480.974

Our AMA:

1. Will evaluate relevant federal legislation related to telemedicine;

2. Urges CMS and other concerned entities involved in telemedicine to fund demonstration projects to evaluate the effect of care delivered by physicians using telemedicine-related technology on costs, quality, and the physician-patient relationship;

3. Urges medical specialty societies involved in telemedicine to develop appropriate practice parameters to address the various applications of telemedicine and to guide quality assessment and liability issues related to telemedicine; (Reaffirmed by CME/CMS Rep. A-96)

4. Encourages the CPT Editorial Board to develop CPT codes or modifiers for telemedical services;

5. Will work with CMS and other payers to develop and test, through these demonstration projects, appropriate reimbursement mechanisms;

6. Will develop a means of providing appropriate continuing medical education credit, acceptable toward the Physician's Recognition Award, for educational consultations using telemedicine; and

7. Will work with the Federation of State Medical Boards and the state and territorial licensing boards to develop licensure guidelines for telemedicine practiced across state boundaries.

(CMS/CME Rep., A-94; Reaffirmation A-01)

Allocation of Privileges to Use Health Care Technologies H-480.988

The AMA (1) affirms the need for the Association and specialty societies to enhance their leadership role in providing guidance on the training, experience and knowledge necessary for the application of specific health care technologies; (2) urges physicians to continue to ensure that, for every patient, technologies will be utilized in the safest and most effective manner by health care professionals; and (3) asserts that licensure of physicians by states must be based on scientific and clinical criteria.

(BOT Rep. F, I-88; Reaffirmed: CME Rep. 8, I-93; Reaffirmed: CME Rep. 2, A-05)

Licensure and Liability for Senior Physician Volunteers D-160.991

Our AMA

1. And its Senior Physician Group will inform physicians about federal and state-based charitable immunity laws that protect physicians wishing to volunteer their services in free medical clinics and other venues

2. Will work with organizations representing free clinics to promote opportunities for physicians who wish to volunteer.

(BOT Rep. 17, A-04)

Alternate Licensure Protocols for IMGs D-255.997

Our AMA will actively support the Florida Medical Association in pursuing legislation that would require the Florida Department of Health to prevent and negate separate criteria for International Medical Graduates to become licensed as Florida physicians.

(Res. 311, A-00)

Eliminating Disparities in Licensure for IMG Physicians D-275.966

Our AMA will advocate and assist the state medical societies to seek legislative action eliminating any disparity in the years of graduate medical education training required for full and unrestricted licensure between IMG and LCME graduates.

(Res. 327, A-08)

Telemedicine and Medical Licensure D-275.967

Our AMA will work with the Federation of State Medical Boards to study how guidelines regulating medical licenses are affected by telemedicine and medical technological innovations that allow for physicians to practice outside their states of licensure.

(Res. 317, A-08)

Depression and Physician Licensure D-275.974

Our AMA will

1. Recommend that physicians who have major depression and seek treatment not have their medical licenses and credentials routinely challenged but instead have decisions about their licensure and credentialing and recredentialing be based on professional performance

2. Make this resolution known to the various state medical licensing boards and to hospitals and health plans involved in physician credentialing and recredentialing.

(Res. 319, A-05)

Arbitrary Exclusion of International Medical Schools Which Impacts Physician Licensure D-275.976

Our AMA will, in close consultation with its IMG Section, work with the Federation of State Medical Boards in its current efforts to study methods to evaluate international medical schools for licensure of their graduates.

(Res. 310, A-05)

Initial State Licensure
D-275.978

Our AMA will work with the Federation of State Medical Boards, state medical societies, state medical boards, and state legislatures, to eliminate the additional graduate medical education requirements imposed on IMGs for an unrestricted license, in the earnest hope of implementing AMA Policy H-275.985.

(Res. 831, I-04)

Simplifying the State Medical Licensure Process
D-275.980

Our AMA Board of Trustees will assign appropriate individuals from within the AMA to work with the Federation of State Medical Boards and keep the AMA membership apprised of the FSMB's actions on developing a standardized medical licensure application, and the individuals assigned by the AMA Board of Trustees regarding the FSMB's work on standardized medical licensure application will report back to the AMA on a yearly basis beginning at the 2005 Annual Meeting, until decided by the Board of Trustees that this is no longer necessary.

(Res. 324, A-04)

Licensure and Liability for Senior Physician Volunteers
D-275.984

Our AMA (1) and its Senior Physician Group will inform physicians about special state licensing regulations for volunteer physicians; and (2) will support and work with state medical licensing boards and other appropriate agencies, including the sharing of model state legislation, to establish special reduced-fee volunteer medical license for those who wish to volunteer their services to the uninsured or indigent.

(BOT Rep. 17, A-04)

Unified Medical License Application
D-275.992

Our AMA will request the Federation of State Medical Boards to examine the issue of a standardized medical licensure application form for those data elements that are common to all medical licensure applications.

(Res. 308, I-01)

Facilitating Credentialing for State Licensure
D-275.994

Our AMA will:

1. Encourage the Federation of State Medical Boards to urge its Portability Committee to complete its work on developing mechanisms for greater reciprocity between state licensing jurisdictions as soon as possible

2. Work with the Federation of State Medical Boards and the Association of State Medical Board Executive Directors to encourage the increased standardization of credentials requirements for licensure, and to increase the number of reciprocal relationships among all licensing jurisdictions

3. Encourage the Federation of State Medical Boards and its licensing jurisdictions to widely disseminate information about the Federation's Credentials Verification Service, especially when physicians apply for a new medical license.

(Res. 302, A-01)

Licensure and Credentialing Issues
D-275.995

Our AMA will:

1. Support recognition of the Federation of State Medical Boards' (FSMB) Credentials Verification Service by all licensing jurisdictions

2. Work jointly with the FSMB to take measures to encourage increased standardization of credentials requirements, and improved portability by increased use of reciprocal relationships among all licensing jurisdictions

3. Communicate, either directly by letter or through its publications, to all hospitals and licensure boards that the Joint Commission on Accreditation of Healthcare Organizations encourages recognition of both the Educational Commission for Foreign Medical Graduates' Certification Verification Service and the AMA's Masterfile as primary source verification of medical school credential; and

4. Encourage the National Commission on Quality Assurance (NCQA) and all other organizations to accept the Federation of State Medical Boards' Credentials Verification Service, the Educational Commission for Foreign Medical Graduates' Certification Verification Service, and the AMA Masterfile as primary source verification of credentials.

(Res. 303, I-00; Reaffirmation A-04)

Response to the Federation of State Medical Boards Recommendations on Licensure
D-275.998

Our AMA will collaborate with other appropriate external groups to develop model state medical licensing legislation or regulations that ensure the public safety.

(Res. 319 , I-98)

State Authority and Flexibility in Medical Licensure for Telemedicine
D-480.999

Our AMA will:

1. Develop a policy regarding the practice of medicine as it relates to the prescribing of prescription-only pharmaceuticals or other therapies via the Internet

2. Continue its opposition to a single national federalized system of medical licensure.

(CME Rep. 7, A-99)

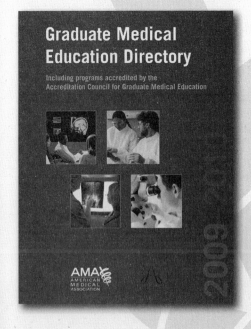

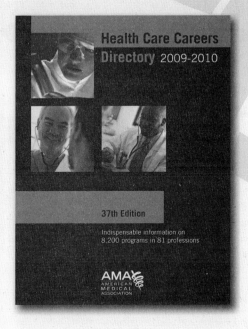

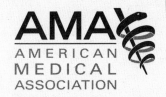

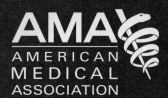
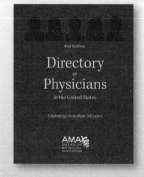
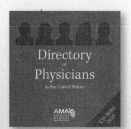
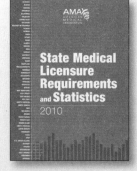
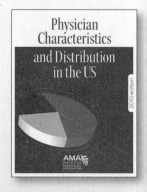